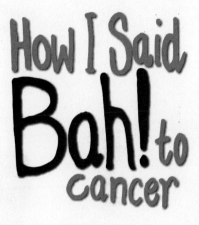

How I Said Bah! to cancer

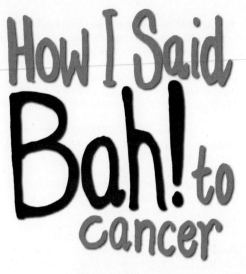

How I Said Bah! to cancer

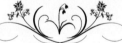

A Guide to Thinking,
Laughing, Living & Dancing
Your Way Through

STEPHANIE BUTLAND
Foreword by **Dr Edward de Bono**

HAY HOUSE
Australia • Canada • Hong Kong • India
South Africa • United Kingdom • United States

First published and distributed in the United Kingdom by:
Hay House UK Ltd, 292B Kensal Rd, London W10 5BE. Tel.: (44) 20 8962 1230;
Fax: (44) 20 8962 1239. www.hayhouse.co.uk

Published and distributed in the United States of America by:
Hay House, Inc., PO Box 5100, Carlsbad, CA 92018-5100. Tel.: (1) 760 431 7695 or
(800) 654 5126; Fax: (1) 760 431 6948 or (800) 650 5115. www.hayhouse.com

Published and distributed in Australia by:
Hay House Australia Ltd, 18/36 Ralph St, Alexandria NSW 2015. Tel.: (61) 2 9669 4299;
Fax: (61) 2 9669 4144. www.hayhouse.com.au

Published and distributed in the Republic of South Africa by:
Hay House SA (Pty), Ltd, PO Box 990, Witkoppen 2068. Tel./Fax: (27) 11 467 8904.
www.hayhouse.co.za

Published and distributed in India by:
Hay House Publishers India, Muskaan Complex, Plot No.3, B-2, Vasant Kunj, New Delhi –
110 070. Tel.: (91) 11 4176 1620; Fax: (91) 11 4176 1630. www.hayhouse.co.in

Distributed in Canada by:
Raincoast, 9050 Shaughnessy St, Vancouver, BC V6P 6E5. Tel.: (1) 604 323 7100;
Fax: (1) 604 323 2600

© Stephanie Butland, 2011

The moral rights of the author have been asserted.

The information given in this book should not be treated as a substitute for professional
medical advice; always consult a medical practitioner. Any use of the information in this
book is at the reader's discretion and risk. Neither the author nor the publisher can be
held responsible for any loss, claim or damage arising out of the use, or misuse, or the
suggestions made or the failure to take medical advice.

A catalogue record for this book is available from the British Library.

ISBN 978-1-84850-591-9

Printed and bound in Great Britain by
TJ International, Padstow, Cornwall.

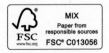

MIX
Paper from
responsible sources
FSC® C013056

For Alan, Ned and Joy,
without whom I would not be possible

Contents

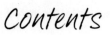

❧ Contents ❧

Contents

❧ Contents ❧

Acknowledgements

It was Jude who coined the phrase 'Bah! to cancer' and, with it, a way for me to think, and cope, and live, and write.

Early and enthusiastic readers of this book included Alan Butland, Libby Turner, Gilly Meek, Denyse Kirkby, Rachel Pearce, Scarlet Long, Emily Medland, Diane Mulholland, Nathalie Giauque, Jen Walshaw, Cynthia Barlow-Marrs, Debby Hornburg, Nicola Kim, Susan Young and Maggie Dana. I'm grateful to them all for their time, comments and re-readings, and in some cases for revisiting painful times for the sake of this book. I'm grateful, too, to Bah! blog readers everywhere, who have been endlessly supportive and encouraging.

In publishing, Jessica Axe pointed me in the right direction. Jude Evans, Scott Pack, Emma Buckley and Nicola Morgan all gave time and advice that moved this book along. They did it with good humour, good grace and as though they like nothing better than reading cancer books on their days off. I'm proud to call them friends.

Jane Smith, Emily Medland, Claire Marriott and Jane Wenham-Jones all contributed to the Blake Friedmann auction on my behalf, helping me to get the Best Agent Ever, Oli Munson. He's a star. So is everyone else at Blake Friedmann, come to that.

The team at Hay House is everything a novice author would want in a publisher: enthusiastic, professional, tireless and kind. Special thanks to my editor, Carolyn Thorne, who made sure that this book remained my book.

☙ Acknowledgements ☙

Andrew Day asked Edward de Bono to write the Foreword for me, when he really should have been getting on with more important things. Edward wrote a generous Foreword, when he probably had better things to do, too. More than that, his simple and elegant approach to thinking has given shape and strength to my life – and this book.

Emily, Nathalie and Susan are a trinity of strength, love and friendship, and have been Bah! book cheerleaders from the start.

Louise Williams had a good feeling, which meant a great deal.

Alan, Ned and Joy have walked every word of this book with me. It wouldn't be in your hand without them. Or without my parents, Michael and Helen Breeze, who taught me that I could do anything if I put my mind to it, and have quietly believed in me all my life.

The people I've mentioned here are people who've helped with this book. Many more have helped me during my dance with cancer. There are too many to name, but I acknowledge you all with every day I am well. Thank you.

I was never going to die from cancer. That hard lump peeping out of the top of my bra was aggressive but it was small enough to be contained, and I was young and strong and otherwise well. All the signs were good. Words like 'lucky' and 'caught in time' were thrown around like rice at a wedding. No, I was never going to die from cancer. But from the beginning, I never planned simply to survive it. Oh no. I was going to say a great big Bah! to it. Please, join in.

Cancer?

Bah!

Foreword

Stephanie has been an excellent trainer of my thinking methods, such as Lateral Thinking™ and Six Thinking Hats®. A really good trainer like Stephanie has to really understand the processes she is teaching.

I am really delighted to hear that Stephanie finds that the positive and creative thinking has been of help to her in her battle with her illness.

It has long been thought that mental attitude and thinking are important in the fight against cancer. Stephanie reports that she has found this to be the case. I congratulate her on this demonstration of this effect. I hope that her experience may also inspire others.

Edward de Bono

Introduction

BAH! TO CANCER

Shortly after surgery, my friend Jude sent me a card. In it she wrote, '... and BAH! TO CANCER' in big letters and everyone who read it, including me, smiled and repeated the phrase out loud: 'Bah! to cancer'. There's something derisive, trivializing about it, and I think that's what I liked. Although I'm not sure that 'Bah!' had ever passed my lips before, it's the sort of word I imagine saying if I got on a train for a long journey and discovered I didn't have a book with me, or arrived for my beach holiday without flip-flops. So, a noise for things that are, ultimately, trivial. Things that deserve a 'Bah!' are annoyances that pass, and are either forgotten or turned into good stories. Over the months following diagnosis with breast cancer, while I blogged and talked about this wretched disease, the Bah! approach crystallized into four elements: thinking, laughing, living, and dancing.

THIS BOOK IS FOR YOU IF ...

This book is for you if you want to say Bah! to cancer, whether you have just stepped onto the floor or are coming to the end of your dance. It tells you what happened to me: what I learned, and the mistakes I think I made. It offers you new ways to think about what is happening in your life. It's full of practical ideas and useful tips about thinking, questioning and behaving in ways to get the best outcome that you can.

This book is for you if someone you love is dancing with cancer. It will give you an insight into what your partner, friend, family member, or colleague might be going through. You will find ideas about how you can support them. You might understand more about the choices that they make. And you might find answers to questions you'd rather not ask them directly.

Whoever you are, I hope that this book will act as guide, information source and friend. I hope it helps you think differently, laugh a little, live well and understand more.

Whoever you are, I wish you well. I wish you very well indeed.

THINKING

When you find that you have a cancer, you step into a world where the physical is king. All manner of machines are used to look at what's lurking under your skin. Your blood is taken, your veins are assessed, people draw on you and paint you with iodine and cut you open. Bits of your body that you used to take for granted – your hair, your nails, your gut, the inside of your nose and mouth – start to behave differently, and bring you worry, and pain. So it's very easy to focus on the body. But, for me, the mind was the part that mattered.

Unless you have a cancer in your brain, your mind is not affected. And the mind is a powerful, powerful thing. Recovering from depression showed me that it's how I *think* about life, not life itself, that could make me happy or wretched. At my first training job with the long-term unemployed, I recognized the power of the self-fulfilling prophesy: everyone who told me that they 'just knew they would never work again' failed to find a job.

Now I work with the mind. Dr Edward de Bono is the world's leading authority on thinking and the teaching of thinking as a skill, and I use his tools for creativity and parallel thinking – I'm one of around 50 Master Trainers in de Bono methods worldwide. In my work, I see again and again how applying a different perspective can instantly unlock a problem or change a decision. So I know that the mind matters.

I've worked with a team of people who simply could not make a decision about filling some senior positions in their organization. Some different thinking tools helped them to see that they were focusing on the wrong problem: not 'Should we promote X or not?' but 'What are we doing in the organization to make sure we have enough good people available to develop and promote?' That session resulted in a complete overhaul of their training and development strategy, with far-reaching effects on company performance as well as a resolution to the original difficulty. On another occasion I worked with a UK Government department trying to make a decision – the problem was that 35 different stakeholders were involved, and each had its own view about how the decision should go to suit its area of interest. A different approach to thinking meant that a decision was reached and a strategy decided in less than two hours. I've also helped a multinational organization decide to restructure and reduce its IT support systems, saving millions – no mean feat when the Director of IT is in the room with his heels dug in so deeply that only his toes are visible sticking up through the carpet! A team using the de Bono thinking strategies will typically see their meeting times reduced by a half, and there will be no argument, no turf-protection, no lengthy anecdotes – only a different way of thinking.

We assume that we think in the same way that we breathe: instinctively, without effort and without anyone needing to teach us to do it. This is true … to a point. Of course you don't need anyone to teach you to breathe. Or do you? If you take swimming lessons, or go on a public speaking course, or learn to sing or practise yoga, the first thing you will need to learn is how to breathe better, because if you breathe better, you will perform better. The same applies to thinking. Yes, you can think … but if you learn some tools for thinking, you'll become much more effective at it. Dr de Bono says that, 'the way we think is not the same as how intelligent we are, in the same way that the power of a car is nothing to do with how well it is driven.' I see this every day in my professional life, and I use it every day in my personal life, too.

So when I was diagnosed with a breast cancer, I listened as I was told what would happen to me; I read leaflet after leaflet about diet and hormones and how to tie a scarf around my newly bald head … But what I was waiting for was someone to mention attitude, or thinking strategies. Surely, I reasoned, the way I think about cancer will be critical to how I cope with it, maybe even to my recovery …? Surely the medical profession, of all people, will know how much thinking matters? But no one ever mentioned thinking. So I applied the de Bono techniques, which I saw succeeding at work: I decided to think differently, knowing that if I changed the thinking, I changed the problem. If I thought effectively, I would find solutions and I would cope better.

But let me say this: In the same way that I don't believe that a rare berry is a cure for cancer, I don't believe that you can 'think yourself better'. Life is not that simple, although there are people who would have you believe that it is. (I'd give them a wide berth if I were you.) And I don't believe that all of the people who have died of cancer would have lived if they had thought different thoughts. But I do believe that you can *choose* what to think about. I do believe that there is potency in the way that we focus our minds. And I believe that my dance with cancer was made easier owing to the way that I chose to think about it.

There's more to this than what's sometimes called 'positive thinking', which, funnily enough, is not a phrase that resonates with positive associations for many people. Maybe that's because it suggests a sort of fingers-in-ears, 'if-I-can't-hear-you-then-it's-not-true' approach to life, which doesn't help anyone much. (Walking around a garden saying 'no weeds, no weeds, no weeds' is not going to win anyone any golden watering cans.)

For me, positive thinking takes real effort. Positive thinking means making active choices about what the mind does. It means choosing to focus on the good news, when there is good news. Positive thinking means stopping a train of thought that is destructive – 'I'm going to die' – and replacing it with one that nurtures – 'I'm going to live.' The brain is a very clever piece of kit, and lots of Very Clever People are still trying to suss out exactly why techniques like this work. But it seems that they *can* work, and it's probably something to do with the way the brain assimilates and processes the information that it's given – and every thought, whether true or false, fact or fiction, is just another piece of information to the brain. Scientists think (although they'd put it in a lot more words than I'm about to) that if you keep thinking about success, your brain sees success as well established, and then goes about trying to make it happen. Mohammed Ali was saying, 'I am the greatest,' for a long time before he was.

USING THIS BOOK

Throughout this book you will find exercises and invitations to 'Bah! thinking'. I might ask you to use your imagination, or make a list, or focus on a word. What I'll ask you to do are things that I've done – or wish I'd done – to make my dance with cancer easier. Most come from my experience with de Bono tools, but some are drawn from NLP (neuro-linguistic programming: the idea that the language we use shapes the way our brains behave), and some from figuring it out as I go along. I've found them helpful, and I sincerely hope that you do, too.

You'll also find that there are extracts from my blog, which I've included to show you what I was experiencing at the time. I've abridged some of them to make them make more sense in their places in this book.

LAUGHING

A sense of humour is the best thing that you can take into cancer with you. Funny stuff happens, even on the darkest days in life. (When my grandmother died, the house was swamped with condolence cards. Two of them were the same. On the day of the funeral, one of my little cousins came in and said excitedly, 'Oooh, look, we've got a swap.') Laughing at them is good for you, physically – unless you've got stitches – and mentally. I got the giggles when a doctor asked me, 'And apart from the cancer, are you in good health?' My mum and I didn't dare look at each other as a nurse due to check my dressings appeared unable to put on a pair of surgical gloves. A doctor writing 'This one' with a felt tip pen on your shoulder, with an arrow drawn down to your breast, before you go into surgery? C'mon, that's hilarious. There are a whole load of oncologist jokes quietly doing the rounds of the bald and pale in waiting rooms around the world. (My favourite: Why are coffins nailed shut? To stop oncologists from getting in and giving you one last dose of chemo to be on the safe side.) I wasn't keeping score, but I'm fairly sure I laughed more than I cried during cancer treatment; it made me feel that life was still good.

LIVING

Life does not stop when cancer arrives, which is an excellent thing. If everyone had sat around looking at me in the manner of Dickensian orphans with TB I'd have been driven up several walls. Parents' evenings, school trips, birthdays, new babies, all keep happening. I was determined to still take part in all of these things, and found that by a clever mix of planning, delegation and lowering my standards a little, I could mostly manage to keep up. So I went to parents' evenings, but I was prepared to opt out after seeing three teachers rather than seven. Everyone got birthday presents, but I spent more time doing online research and less time in shops. When I realized I wasn't going to be able to knit a baby gift to the deadline, I gave the yarn and pattern to my mum and she did it for me. (She still hasn't forgiven me for the miles of picot trim.)

I was determined to keep working through my dance with cancer: I didn't want to sit around Having Cancer for months, and I love my job. So I worked fewer days and travelled less, but I kept my professional identity, and that made me feel alive, even if there were days when I overdid it and felt half-dead as a consequence.

Then there was my social life. I love going to the theatre. I love eating out, and sitting round a table with friends talking into the night. I love walking, whether it's the south bank of the Thames in London or a quiet forest footpath. I tried to keep on doing what I love. It didn't make any sense to me not to. But there were compromises. When we went to the theatre, I'd rest in the afternoon. We ate out close to home so there wasn't a tube journey to contend with. There were days when I couldn't walk as far as the post office on the corner, but on days when I had more energy I walked round the park or to a café where I could have a rest before I walked back again.

BAH! THINKING

What matters?

It's easy to let cancer take over your life. Here's a simple strategy to make sure you keep it in its place.

- Make a list of all the things that you like to do. It doesn't have to be an Official And Admirable Hobby. Sex, soap operas, scuba diving, it doesn't matter. If you like it, write it down.

- Now write a number next to each. If you 'can't live without it,' it's a 10. A 1 would be 'maybe I don't really enjoy doing this as much as I thought I did.'

- Now take a fresh sheet of paper. Write 'I will keep on ...' at the top and write the five pastimes that scored the highest underneath. Post the list somewhere you will see it every day.

- Now do whatever you need to do to make sure that these important parts of your life still happen. You may need to make some substitutions: if you're not going to be able to scuba-dive, at least make sure you can swim.

There have been days during my dance with cancer when what I really felt like doing was lying under the duvet, working myself into a state about all of the terrible cancer-related things that could happen. On days like that it's hard to get up and dressed and put some lip-gloss on and go to the library for another armful of Agatha Christies, but it's the positive choice. And, just as staying in bed makes everything worse, that little trip to the library starts you on an upward curve. The exercise helps your body to process the chemotherapy drugs that are in it. The fresh air invigorates. Watching a little girl, dressed entirely in pink, gravely manoeuvre her pram full of teddy bears up a kerb, and exchanging a look of shared amusement with her mother, takes your attention away from yourself for just a minute.

Stay in the world, as much as you can.

DANCING

As soon as I started to tell people that I had a cancer, the encouragement began to tumble in. I was exhorted to 'fight' and 'beat it' and was assured that I would 'win the battle'. As someone who has never hit anyone in her life – saying 'Bah!' is about as violent as I get – all of this fighting talk made me a little scared. And I hated the idea that people who had died from cancer had somehow 'lost the fight'. Still, there was a lot going on, so I didn't think too much about it.

Later, after surgery, I emailed a knitting designer to tell her that making her beautiful moebius patterns had given me just the right combination of stimulation and comfort. She replied and her email contained the phrase, 'my own dance with cancer'. *Dancing with cancer.* I rolled the phrase round my mouth, enjoying the feel of it, the way the words circled each other. And then I started to think about what the phrase meant, and I knew that I could ditch the battle metaphors once and for all.

A dance needs two people, so 'dancing with cancer' suggests a kind of equality. I like that better than thinking of little tiny me battling with cancer, which everyone knows is very big and very scary. And I like the idea that I am not being dragged and hauled and pummelled by cancer. In a battle, cancer could win, and if it did, where would I be? In a dance, I have much more power over the outcome. Most importantly, though, I'm unlikely to die of dancing. And one day, the music will stop and I will step off the dance floor. I might be weary, I might well have the odd blister, I might find that my life is different owing to the unscheduled dance, but I will be alive.

There's a broader point behind the dance metaphor, and that is that there is power, such power, in the words we choose and use. If anyone ever described me as a 'cancer victim' or 'cancer sufferer', I either corrected or ignored them, because language like that really brought me down. I have never referred to myself as having cancer – it has always been 'a' cancer, singular. And I have certainly never said 'my cancer'. I have no intention of owning such a tedious, nasty little thing, thank you all the same.

BAH! THINKING

Your language of cancer

The power of the language around cancer is completely yours. Take a look at this list and see which description resonates with you, or add one of your own:

- a person with cancer

- someone dancing with cancer

- someone living with cancer

- someone living with cancer, for now

- a person surviving cancer

- someone battling cancer

- someone fighting cancer

- someone being treated for cancer

- a person triumphing over cancer

- a person beating cancer

- someone getting rid of a cancer

Whatever you decide suits you, use it with everyone, and use it without apology. (My friends and family now talk about my dance with cancer as though 'dance' is the most natural way in the world of describing it.)

Diagnosis: In the beginning was the lump

HOW IT WAS

I found a lump in my right breast toward the end of September 2008.

Now, don't go thinking that I had some kind of breast-examination regime in the manner of a proper grown-up. I am the kind of person who, after buying shoes reduced from £100 to £50 in a sale, thinks that she has £50 to spend. At 37, I had only just got round to starting a pension. The reason I found the lump was that I could see it. I was walking past the mirror on my way to the shower, the light caught a distended area at the top of my right breast, and I thought 'Hmph! That spoils my line.' And that's how my dance with cancer began.

But let's start at the moment before I walked past the mirror: Let's start from me, walking upstairs, thinking about a good hot shower and pyjamas and then sitting down with my husband, Alan, to do a crossword or talk about what we might do next weekend. If I'd stopped and thought about my life then, as I took off my shoes and looked around our bedroom and wondered why it never stayed tidy for more than 10 minutes, I'd have thought myself pretty lucky. My first 37 years had meandered along, without much of a plan, or much of a purpose, but despite this I had somehow acquired more than enough to make me more than happy. My second marriage was a delight every day, and my children from my first marriage, at 12 and 14, were growing into young adults I was proud to know and love. My career as a trainer was going well, I loved working, and I also loved the fact that I didn't need to be working all of the time. I was running a cake business and doing a psychology degree in my 'spare' time. And I had finally shaken off the depression that had stalked me for more than a decade. Life was good.

But I didn't stop and think about my life and how much there was in it, because ... well, who does, when the going is good?

I've met people who have told me that when they found lumps in their body, they Just Knew It Was Cancer. I didn't. I knew it was a lump, obviously. And I knew that there was no history of breast cancer in my family. I knew that I was 'too young' to have breast cancer and I knew that most breast lumps are harmless/caused by the menstrual cycle/come and go. (I'd obviously been paying more attention to posters in doctors' waiting rooms than I'd realized.) So, I didn't think the lump was a cancer. But I didn't think it *wasn't* cancer, either. That was a pretty big step for me. The first, as it happened, in a whole series of pretty big steps.

Edward de Bono: A White Hat and a lump

One of the most well-known de Bono tools is called the Six Thinking Hats®, where each of six different coloured (notional) hats represents a different type of thinking. So, when a group embarks on Yellow Hat thinking, everyone will be looking for benefits in the given situation. Black Hat thinking is for risks, Green Hat for creativity. And White Hat is for information: What do we know? What do we need to know? I'm often asked to work with teams who simply cannot make a decision about something, and believe that the problem is that the arguments for and against are too finely balanced, so they need a bit of specialist help (me). And in, ooh, about 126 out of 129 of those situations, the problem is something else entirely. There might be a lot of assumptions and suppositions clouding the decision-making process, but what almost always works is focusing back on what we know, and what we need to know. Most often, the difficulty is a missing critical piece of information that has been overlooked. Find out what it is – by asking the right questions, by taking out the speculation and opinion and guesswork – and the decision makes itself. So I know how much information matters.

Now, it doesn't take a genius to see the problem with a lump. What do we know? It's a lump. What do we need to know? Whether the lump is a cancer.

The early stage of diagnosis is, potentially, a wretched place full of dark imaginings and wobbly lipped, fearful faces. (Even if you don't tell anyone, your reflection ain't going to get a sparklingly enthusiastic response from a magic mirror.) And it's hard to handle. I found a couple of thinking techniques helped me through the days and weeks of cold hands and sharp needles:

First, I saw every test as one more piece of crucial information that was going to move things on, one way or the other. (And, over those next few weeks, it did feel as though every man and his dog was having a feel and a poke and a good look. Fortunately dogs do not have opposable thumbs, so they can't wield needles.)

Second, I limited the time I spent thinking about the lump.

TESTING, TESTING: COLLECTING THE DATA

1. GP

I'm a fan of my GP. He always treats me like an intelligent woman who should have a say in the treatment of her own health. That shouldn't be unusual, but on the few occasions when I've needed to see a doctor who wasn't Dr Adeyemi, I've found that it is. Dr A asked me about family history and other risk factors, which were minimal, unless you come from the school of thought that says underwired bras, underarm deodorants and generally being born in the later stages of the twentieth century cause cancer. Dr A referred me to the Breast Unit at St George's Hospital in Tooting, just to be on the safe side. This seemed sensible to me and I was happy to go along.

2. Breast Unit

Less than a week later, Joe, a nurse practitioner at St George's, diagnosed the lump as 'probably a cyst or a fatty deposit' (nice) but sent me for an ultrasound scan and mammogram anyway, and then stabbed me with a needle. (It's called a fine-needle biopsy, took about five seconds and a bit of jiggling – by the needle, not me – and didn't hurt a bit.) I discovered afterwards that these three tests are accepted best practice for the examination of shifty looking breast lumps. None of them felt like much of a big deal. The ultrasound involves being smeared in cold gel and having a reader attached to a monitor passed over both breasts while the technician captures the images. (Everyone always apologizes that the gel is cold. Why don't they just WARM IT UP? It's not like there are no radiators in hospitals.) The mammogram means having the breast squished between two glass plates in a variety of ways. It's a bit uncomfortable but the comedy factor more than makes up for the discomfort, in my view. And the fine-needle biopsy really was over before I knew it.

3. Biopsy Suite

A week or so after the three tests I got a letter, to the effect of it would be a good idea to have an ultrasound-guided biopsy just in case. (Nobody said just in case *what* yet, but we all knew. I started to get a bit wobbly at this point.) The biopsy would also take in an irregular area in the left breast identified by the ultrasound.

The ultrasound-guided biopsy was where it started to get serious in terms of The Word No One Had Yet Mentioned. (There was a nurse there whose only job seemed to be to hold my hand.) This set of biopsies was a bit more involved than the earlier brief stabbing. First, local anaesthetic. Then, incisions – I wasn't allowed to look but I was aware of the mopping up of blood. Then there were four goes each side with a spring-loaded hollow needle. The part of me that enjoys medical documentaries found this interesting. Once the radiographer has found the area to take a sample from (there was some shoving to get to that point), there is a loud click, which is the sound of the spring-loaded part of the needle popping out and in again and taking a cylinder of tissue with it. The tissue then goes into a little basket and can go to the lab to be sliced and examined.

The incisions were covered up with steri-strips and I was dismissed before the anaesthetic wore off. (Very clever, hospital people.) At home, the bruising and aching started, and the whole of the afternoon was pretty miserable. I think I watched TV, which I would never normally do during the day, although, as it happened, this was good training for what was to come.

BAH! THINKING

Limiting thinking time

You have power over what you think about, and you can control how you think. Try any (or all) of these techniques to help you deal with this uncertain time.

1. Set aside five minutes, morning and evening (but not immediately before bed), to think about the possibility of cancer. Use a clock to measure out the minutes. For five minutes, worry, cry, imagine the worst. When your five minutes are done, stop. Take a deep breath, straighten your spine, and go and do something else. When your thoughts wander back toward the diagnostic process, gently remind your brain that this is not the time. Wait until the time comes again.

2. Find a quiet place, take a deep breath, and write down exactly what it is that you're afraid of. Maybe it is as simple – and dreadful – as 'I'm afraid of dying.' Maybe it's more complicated: fear of pain, of letting others down, of changes that will come if you are diagnosed with a cancer. Whatever it is, write it down, as fully and explicitly as you can. This will hurt. It will be difficult. But when it's done, it's done. Read what you've written, close your notebook and go on your way. I'm not suggesting that doing this will have made your fears vanish. But there's a good chance that getting them out of your heart and onto the page will make them easier to cope with, and give them less power to stalk you.

3. Work out when you're most worried, and do something to avoid or change that situation. If you find yourself catastrophizing while you have a bath, take a shower. If walking home is when your thoughts become unbearable, listen to music or an audio book as you go.

4. If there is someone you are regularly talking to about your fears and worries, ask them to help you to control your thoughts. This might be by setting a time-limit on conversations, or being clear about what you want from the conversation. So you might say, 'I really want to just get everything off my chest and for you to listen,' or, 'Would you please help me to work out what I will do if I am diagnosed?' or even, 'Will you stop me if I start repeating myself or going round in circles?'

By now, I'd told friends Louise, Scarlet and Jude, who were all supportive in their different ways. Lou is the glass-half-empty to my glass-half-full, so she looked anxious, just as I expected she would. And she lost her mother to cancer, so she has good reason to cut her eyes at the c-word. Both of Scarlet's parents have danced with cancer, so she had a lot of practical knowledge to offer. I don't remember telling Jude about finding the lump and having tests, but I do remember a Sunday afternoon in a coffee shop with her, talking about what the results might be.

It was when I called the hospital, because I hadn't had either a letter telling me all was well, or an appointment to come in, and was told, 'Oh, yes, we do need to see you,' that I decided it was time to tell my parents what was going on. I hated the idea of telling them such Big News (or Possibly Big News) over the phone, and had put off talking to them because they were coming to visit the next week. But their visit was going to be after my Getting The News appointment and I hated the idea of telling them as soon as they arrived. (I thought about my Uncle Alan who, when we were children, used to get us in a headlock and ask whether we wanted long illness or sudden death.)

So, I called at a time when I thought they would both be there. They weren't, but my dad was on his way home. 'Do you want to start?' Mum asked, and I said, 'I found a lump in my breast just before you went on holiday and I've had lots of tests and I'm going back to the hospital for results next week but it's not looking very good.' (I said it just like that, with no punctuation at all.) She said 'Oh, no,' very quietly, and I know she was thinking about the terrible time one of our in-laws had the year before, when she had a mastectomy, chemotherapy and radiotherapy. I took her through all of the tests that I'd had and what various people had said at the different stages, and I felt like the world's worst daughter.

A fortnight later and it was back to the Breast Clinic for the results. Alan was meeting me at the hospital, and as I walked down the road I had a moment of clarity: I was going to be told that this was a cancer. I was shaky and afraid. I met Alan and, as we headed into the clinic, I noticed something that looked like 'pre-operative' highlighted next to my name on the receptionist's sheet.

We didn't have to wait long. Joe called me and I went into a consulting room. Alan stayed in the waiting area. I'm not sure why. Maybe we were just obedient in the face of institutionalization – he wasn't called. Maybe it was the last part of me grasping at a quick in-and-out, 'that's all fine, Mrs Butland, nothing to worry about' type consultation. Anyway. It all got a bit Pinteresque. Here's the script.

[STEPHANIE/ME enters a small, stuffy office, which has a tiny window high up in the wall. There's a door from the clinic waiting area and two other doors adjoining consulting rooms within. JOE, the nurse practitioner, is already in the room. There's a box of tissues and a fat blue file on the desk.]

JOE: (kindly, looking ME straight in the eye) We have your results, Stephanie, and there is a cancer in your right breast.

ME: OK. Right (looks down at breast, as if for confirmation; maybe a thumbs up, 'Hi, it is me after all,' from the lump)

(Mr MOKBEL enters from one of the side rooms and sits behind the desk.)

JOE: This is Mr Mokbel, one of our consultant surgeons. [To MR MOKBEL] I've just told Stephanie that there is a cancer in her right breast. (To STEPHANIE) I'm so sorry. I really thought it was nothing.

ME: Shall I get my husband in?

JOE: Of course.

[ALAN enters and sits down. General greetings and introductions.]

ME: (to ALAN) I do have a cancer in my right breast. (To JOE) Which presumably means that the left side is OK?

(JOE and MR MOKBEL exchange a look.)

JOE: Well …

MR MOKBEL: We know there is a cancer in your right breast. We think it is quite small and we have caught it early. We need to remove the lump.

ME: Not the breast?

MR MOKBEL: The lump only. And at the same time we will examine the lymph nodes under your arm to see whether the cancer is there. If it is, we will take out the nodes.

ME: (holding ALAN's hand, probably quite tightly) Not the breast?

MR MOKBEL: Not the breast. (A small part of my brain hangs up some bunting. I have been bosomy for 25 years or so and not ready to stop now.)

ME: Good. That's something.

MR MOKBEL: On the left side, there is a small group of cells that don't look normal, but may not be cancerous. We would like to take them out so we can examine them properly.

ME: (crying a little) [Everyone makes sympathetic noises, including CHARMAINE, the Macmillan nurse, who has come in unnoticed at some point] No, it's not that, it's just that ... my mum will be so upset.

MR MOKBEL: The prognosis is excellent. We have caught this very early, and you are young and in good health. [Someone asks about what happens next. I'd like it to have been ALAN, as he doesn't seem to have said anything yet, although he was doing stalwart hand-holding and eye contact.]

It all goes a bit blurry after that. Alan and I were ushered off to talk to the Macmillan nurse about what would happen in more detail. We talked about who to tell, how to tell them, and the possibilities of what the treatment would be like (which turned out, by and large, to be much worse than they actually were). It was mostly a monologue on the part of the nurse – she seemed to be covering all of the bases that she thought we might be thinking about. I mostly sat and wondered how it was that I came to be sitting in a wicker chair in a white-painted cupboard listening to someone tell me how tired and ill I was going to get, and how emotionally erratic/borderline psychotic everyone needed to prepare for me to be. We came away with a whole lot of leaflets. I tried to avoid the Cupboard of Tears after that.

Alan and I agreed, on the way home, that this was not the end of the world. We agreed that it was 'a cancer' rather than Cancer, and that we would encourage everyone else to think of it that way. We immediately told Mum and Dad, Lou, Scarlet and Jude. Dad said, 'Well, we'll just have to get on with it,' in the way that he would have done if the shed had blown over and had to be rebuilt, and I felt completely safe, because there's no shed in the universe that my dad couldn't fix.

Then we decided we needed a drink, and as the only thing chilled in the house was a bottle of champagne, we drank that.

Very nice it was, too.

A change in perspective

One of the most important things I have learned from Edward de Bono's methods is that it's easy to focus in on a problem, be overwhelmed by the problem and forget the context of the problem, when knowing what the context is might make solving the problem easier, or at least give you a clearer sense of how big the problem is. (I'm not saying that cancer is not a problem. Just that its context – the bigger picture – is a clever body and a broader life.) When I remembered this, one morning after a long night – my dreams, always vivid, had taken sinister twists, full of dark corridors and people who wouldn't talk to me, and a locked room that everyone was scared of – I came up with this visualization. It helped me. I hope it helps you.

BAH! THINKING

A visualization for when you are diagnosed with a cancer

Sit somewhere quiet and close your eyes. Deliberately slow your breathing. Breathe quietly until you feel a rhythm to your breath.

Now, think about all of the things that your body has done. Think about all of the miles it has carried you. Maybe it has borne you children. Maybe it has climbed you to high places, or run you long distances. Think of the hands it has held, the breaths it has taken, the many times it has stretched in the morning, ready to propel you through another day. Think of the things your body has recovered from. Think about how brilliant your body is, and have confidence in what it can do.

Think about how strong you are, and how clever, to be able to do all of the things that you do with so little conscious thought.

Feel how much power there is in your body. Feel full of that power. Feel unassailable. Feel strong. Breathe and enjoy the feeling.

Smile.

Open your eyes.

Do this as often as you need to.

WHAT CANCER IS

The word 'cancer' comes from the Greek *karkinos*, meaning 'crab'. It's thought that the name was first used by the Roman physician Galen, who saw that malignant tumours spread their 'claws' in all directions, and cleaved tightly to the body no matter what you did to try to get the little buggers off.

Normal cells have their own death programmed into their DNA – a process called *apoptosis*. A cancer cell mutates, replicates quickly, and doesn't die. Once cancer cells exist in the body, they take over the body's resources in order to feed and grow, so that the body can no longer function as it should.

Cancer grades and stages

Cancer is measured in grades and stages. Cancer grading varies according to cancer type, but is usually numerical and indicates how fast-growing the cancer is. For breast cancer the grades are 1–3, with 1 being the slowest.

Cancer stages run from I to IV. As with grading, the definition of the stage differs according to the type of cancer, so a stage II breast cancer is different to a stage II liver cancer. But, broadly speaking, stage I means small and localized, and stage IV means you're unlikely to need to buy anything with the word 'durable' on it.

Stages are defined by the 'TNM' classification system, where T describes the size of the tumour and how much tissue it has affected, N is for 'node' and describes lymph node involvement, and M is for 'metastasis' – the spread of cancer to other areas of the body. So, where a tumour is classified as a T1 (teeny), and there are no lymph nodes involved (L0) and no metastasis (M0), you're looking at stage I.

Staging and grade can change after surgery. Before surgery (the clinical stage), despite the wonders of medical science and all of its pokey diagnostic things, there's a degree of speculation about what exactly is going on in your body. Once the tumour is out (the pathological stage), people with microscopes, white coats and a level of attention to detail that I could only ever dream of can examine the cancer tissue and provide more information. Before surgery I thought I had a stage I grade 3 cancer. After surgery it was revised up to a stage II grade 3. I liked the first one better.

Knowing: the White Hat again

Once you have a diagnosis, White Hat thinking comes into its own. Information matters, and there's a whole lot of it about. You can read facts, research, medical opinion, advice, personal stories and statistics. You can talk to others and ask questions. And so you can find out what you need to know. You can make decisions about what will help you and what will not. You can decide when to question medical expertise and when to take it and cling to it for dear life.

Before I had surgery, I was given a leaflet about anaesthesia, which gave me some facts and statistics, and also said that before my operation I would be able to 'discuss options with my anaesthetist and we would decide together what would be best for me'. Now, my knowledge of anaesthetics consisted of what I'd just read in the leaflet. The anaesthetist's knowledge was based on at least a decade of training and experience. If she had told me to lie down while she sprinkled me with sleepy dust, I'd have done as I was told. But there have been other times – when the chemotherapy side effects were about as much fun as queuing in a hailstorm to have a tooth extracted, for example – when asking all of the questions I could think of helped me to make decisions that made an impact on my treatment.

BAH! THINKING 🦅

What do you need to know?

It's a good idea to ask a lot of questions. Here are some to get you started. You will probably have more.

1. **What type of cancer is it? What does that mean?**
   Cancer is not just cancer. There are types within types. So, I had invasive ductal carcinoma, which is also known as 'no special type' breast cancer. (Kick a girl while she's down, why don't you?) 'Invasive' means the cancer has spread outside the ducts of the breast, and 'carcinoma' is a medical word for cancer, a bit like 'this might be a little bit uncomfortable' is a medical way of saying 'this would be a good time to find a stick to bite on.'

2. **What is the stage and grade of the cancer?**

3. **What types of treatments are available?**
   Medical professionals will often get together before seeing you and discuss and decide your treatment. On one level, this is great: the combined wisdom of a surgeon, an oncologist and a specialist nurse practitioner is unlikely to outweigh that of the newly diagnosed. But the downside is that you, as the patient, might be presented with a course of treatment that seems like the *only* one, and you might want to at least know what other options you have.

4. **Why do you think that <recommended treatment> is the best course of action?**
   Again, it's worth asking the question, partly because it will help you to understand what's going on, and partly because I can guarantee that within a week someone will have said to you something along the lines of, 'My Auntie Gwen had exactly the same as what you've got and she was told that surgery wouldn't help.' The person will then look at you expectantly. The more you know, the more likely you are to be able to (a) explain why your treatment might not be the same as Auntie Gwen's, and (b) not lie awake at night wondering why you are having a treatment

that Auntie Gwen's oncology team dismissed. (Don't forget to also (c) remove the number of this insensitive idiot from your phone.)

5.   If I had been diagnosed at another hospital, or by another person, would the recommended treatment be the same? Your team is – understandably – likely to suggest only what it can deliver. It's worth checking to see whether that would differ elsewhere.

6.   When will I be treated?
     I found, over and over, that teeny details like dates were routinely not given to me. (I would get a letter, at some point.) So I would have lots of people to call, explaining that I might not be able to do X but I didn't know yet. Then I had to call them again when I did have an appointment, but for the few days between we'd all be in limbo, and I had double the number of calls to make.

7.   What are the hospital targets for treatment?
     I know people who have been panicked by the fact that surgeons want to operate immediately: they haven't had a chance to plan, to organize, to get used to the idea before they're counting backwards from 10 and it's all going a bit woozy after eight. In some cases, yes, if you have a tumour the size of a wombat pressing on your heart it is a matter of life or death and if the op has to be tomorrow, it has to be tomorrow. More likely, the operation does have to be done, but it could be that you are being pressed to go in on the 22nd rather than the 26th because the 26th falls outside the hospital targets set for treatment. And if it's your four-year-old's birthday on the 24th, well, I think you're entitled to know why the 22nd matters so much, and make your decision about which date suits you accordingly.

8. What else needs to happen before treatment takes place?
   You might need to go to assessment clinics. You might need to have wires inserted under ultrasound and local anaesthetic to guide the surgeon to the right place. If you have a history of heart or lung trouble, you may need CT scans, echocardiograms, X-rays.

9. Who will do my operation?
   I just think it's nice to know. The person on the other end of the scalpel could be saving your life. But then again, I read the badges of the people who scan my groceries and thank them by name. So it might just be me.

10. Could you please explain exactly what will happen during the treatment?
    Obviously, skip this one if you'd prefer, but I like to know what's going on with my body, especially if I'm going to be asleep and miss important stuff.

11. What can I do to help ensure the best outcome?
    You might choose to take the approach that you are now in the hands of the hospital and they are, for the duration, the boss of you. However, my guess is that people who do that end up in a worse state than people who take a bit of responsibility.

12. How long will I stay in hospital?
    Unless you live a family-free, employment-free, friend-free life, you need to know the answer to this so you can plan.

13. How long will it be before I can drive/lift my child/take a bath/return to work?

14. How will we know if the <type of treatment> has been successful?
    Obviously, one answer to this question is, 'If you are still alive in 40 years'. But there will be other ways of measuring.

15. When will we reassess the treatments that I need?
    Asking questions like this mark you out as someone who will be looking out for herself. That can't do any harm.

16. What would happen if we did nothing?
    Know thine enemy.

17. What support services do you offer/know of?
    I found that there were places I could go for support/massages/reflexology/to meet other people dancing with cancer. I usually found out about them because a friend of a friend whose mum had a breast cancer would send me an email that began with the words, 'You probably already know this, but ...' When I mentioned these places back at the hospital, the reaction was generally, 'Oh, yes, I've heard that place is good.' So it wasn't that the staff didn't know, it's just that in the hurly-burly of getting someone onto the cancer conveyor belt, it wasn't mentioned. (It was probably in the leaflets.)

18. What can I do if I have more questions about this?
    While I was at the hospital it was pretty easy to talk to medical staff and find the answers to my questions. But once I'd left the building it was quite another matter. Staff weren't there to answer their phones, or pick up their voicemail. Clinics were closed on Fridays, presumably because Friday is the day of the week where no one has cancer. So it's worth getting email addresses, or bleep numbers. I'm not suggesting that you get the on-call oncologist out of bed at 1 a.m. on a Sunday to ask them if they think another glass Rioja is a good idea, but I do think you need to know how to get hold of people if you need to.

HOW TO HELP: What to say when someone you know is going through diagnosis

1. Do you want me to come with you?

2. I hope it's nothing.

3. Even if it is nothing, this must be pretty traumatic for you.

4. How are you feeling?

5. What happens next? How can I help/support you with that?

At this stage, that is really all I think you can do. But don't underestimate the power of doing it.

🌱 🌱 🌱

Out there: A lot of difficult conversations, quite fast

MANAGING THE CAMPAIGN

Everyone else had to be told I had a cancer, but it was going to be like toppling a line of dominos. My children, Ned and Joy, needed to know, but so did their dad. I wanted them to hear it from me, so I had to tell him at a time when he wouldn't see the children before I did, as it wasn't fair to ask him not to say anything. I had to let colleagues and clients know as soon as possible so that I could reschedule work, and there were some friends who I knew would tell others so I tried to work out a little telephone tree that would make sure everyone would hear it from someone appropriate. There were people who I wanted to tell in person, people I would have to tell over the phone because they lived too far away to meet up with, people who I knew would not be offended by an email. (I didn't text anyone to tell them.) There were people who Alan or my mum could tell, and people who I wanted to hear the news from me. There were people who I knew had cancer 'previous', and people with little or no experience of the disease, and they all needed to be told in the right way.

de Bono on structure

Something that people often report when they've started working with the de Bono tools is that they didn't realize how unstructured their thinking had been before. Our thoughts buzz around in our heads like bluebottles round a bin, and we are so busy with the content of our thinking that we forget about the overall direction. Our brains are easily distracted. They are the equivalent of a tourist in Paris for the first time, following a tour guide for a little while until another one catches their attention, then following the new one instead. If you take that approach to sightseeing then you might get intimately acquainted with Montmartre, but you're unlikely to get as far as the Eiffel Tower. So the more structure we give our thinking, the better we get at both thinking and communicating our thoughts.

de Bono and the Red Hat

Red Hat thinking is all about gut feel, instinct and emotion: what your instinct is telling you *right this moment*. So Red Hat thinking changes. In my work with Six Thinking Hats® it's fascinating to see how strongly feelings dictate our responses without us even noticing – it's easy to believe that what we feel is what is true – and how the simple action of separating and limiting Red Hat thinking makes it easier to manage, and utilize, our feelings and instincts.

Red Hat doesn't call for explanation or justification – it's the simple expression of how we feel about something, here and now. Most people's immediate Red Hat instinct to the word 'cancer' is not going to be a positive one. In fact, I asked a group of people – none of whom, to my knowledge, had had a cancer – to write down three words they thought of when they heard the c-word. No prizes for guessing that 'scary' and 'death' came out near the top, with 'bald' a close third. So the difficulty with telling people that I had a cancer was going to be managing things so that those emotions could be let out, without dominating everything.

THE CONVERSATIONS

Alan and I worked out the order, then the formula

People who regularly give bad news – the police, medics, HR people – are trained to be very good at it. They give the facts as quickly and simply as they can, they allow people time to absorb what they've said, and then they find out what needs to be done next, from the reaction of the person they are talking to. We tried to do the same. It seemed disrespectful to do otherwise. And I think we were aware, even then, even if we hadn't completely articulated it, that the way we told others would influence the way they supported us. We had to get it right.

'Smile, and the world smiles with you,' someone once said, and during the 'telling everyone' time I also found that 'Tell people you have a cancer in quite a positive way and everyone will be positive back; tell them in a teary way and they'll cry and it will all seem worse' was equally true, although it may not have scanned as well.

Actually, it wasn't difficult, as I mostly felt smiley. My Red Hat feeling about cancer was, essentially, 'Phew! caught it in time!' Although the cancer, when removed, would show itself to be stage II in a flattering outfit, at the time we thought it was stage I: tiny and really not worth worrying about. So I was confident about my end of the conversations. And most of the people I told were calm and caring and made me feel secure in my recovery and sure of their support. Apart from the moment when they were absorbing the news, and their Red Hat instinct dominated, and their eyes, just for a blink of time, were wreathed in pity and horror. Everyone had that. But it always passed. And having a structure to the conversations about cancer helped to make that happen.

BAH! THINKING

Planning ahead

Before you start telling people that you are dancing with cancer, think about how you are going to do it. Write down a list of information that you want to cover and what the outcome of the conversation should be. If there are any bits that you will find difficult to say, or might forget, write down some phrases that you can look at and read. I went into every conversation with a note saying, 'I'm not going to die!' as I knew that's where the mind leaps to when cancer is mentioned – but because I was really clear in my own mind that I wasn't going to die, I was afraid I'd forget to give others this reassurance.

Before you pick up the phone, think about the person at the other end. Around 6 p.m. might be a good time for you to make calls, but if your friend has two toddlers, it's unlikely that 6 p.m. is the best time for her. Try to avoid calling people who you know will be anxious late in the evening.

The more you can help people to hear the news well, the easier it will be for you.

Here's a typical conversation with me in November 2008:

Me: Hello. How are you?

Them: (something along the lines of) I'm fine, thanks. How are you?

Me: I'm fine, but I'm calling to let you know some not-so-good news. I've just been diagnosed with a breast cancer.

Them: (something along the lines of) Oh, I'm sorry.

Me: (quickly, before they can start catastrophizing or panicking or asking questions and taking me away from what I need to say) Thank you. It's a very small cancer and they think that it has been caught very early. I'm going to need surgery and radiotherapy and maybe chemotherapy, but I'm feeling very positive, and so are the doctors. None of us thinks there is any chance of me dying of this, so I'm just planning to get through it with the minimum hassle and get back to my life, really.

I wanted to be sure that I'd got over the points that (1) I had a breast cancer, (2) it was small, (3) it had been caught early, (4) I wasn't dying and (5) I was being positive and calm about it. I also hoped that, subconsciously, the fact that I talked about 'having a cancer' (singular) rather than 'having cancer' would have an impact.

Not in front of the children

The conversation that I dreaded was the one with my children. At 14 and 12, Ned and Joy seemed to me to be at the worst possible age to be told that their mother had a cancer. Any younger and they may not have understood the implications. Any older and they might have had the opportunity to develop some coping strategies for crises. As it was, they'd led a life mostly sheltered from unpleasantness. Their father Jason and I divorced when they were very small, and of course that had a big impact, but they had two parents who got on, lived round the corner from each other, and who they both saw regularly. When Alan became part of the family he'd worked hard to make it as easy as possible for us all, although having a step-parent had its challenges. They had lost one grandparent, who they hadn't seen very much of, and their Granny had had lung cancer, and survived it. Mostly, plain sailing.

The day after diagnosis – which happened to fall in the middle of half-term – Ned and Joy were due back from their dad's. Jason was at work, so I'd called him there and told him the news. He was shocked, but he pledged support, and he was as good as his word. (He still is.) Joy asked, 'What are we doing today?' and my heart got heavier. The three of us sat down together. I remember that moment – the moment before I said the words – as a sort of slow-motion heartbreak. Ned and Joy were both looking at me expectantly, and there was no fear or anxiety in either of them, and I knew that what I said next – and no matter how positively I said it, and no matter how clear I was, to me and to them, that this was no more than a health blip, a minor annoyance in our family history – would shift their world on its axis. I knew that, after this conversation, life would divide into 'before Mum had a cancer' and 'after Mum had a cancer'. I knew that next time I said, 'Come and sit down,

I need to talk to you about something', they wouldn't be as relaxed and unconcerned as they were now.

I said, 'I have no idea how to say this to you,' and then I said, 'I've just found out that I have a breast cancer. It's very small and it's not a problem ...' and then I dwindled. Joy cried and threw herself into my arms. Ned held my hand and looked worlds at me. I don't think I've ever been so sad. I wasn't distressed, or upset, or tearful. There was just some part of me that was acknowledging the terribleness of what had happened in those quiet words.

(Some weeks previously, I'd had a conversation with my friend Louise, in which I'd airily opined that if I did have a cancer and die from it, I didn't much mind because I'd had a marvellous life and everyone, including my children, would get on just fine without me. She'd suggested that just maybe, actually, they'd be devastated and I was possibly only saying that because I was protecting myself from that knowledge. If I hadn't figured out that she was right then, I had now.)

We talked about what was going to happen, and Ned still reminds me from time to time that I said, 'Absolutely nothing around here is going to change.' Little did I know. But I wanted them to feel – as I felt, fiercely – that they would still have their mother, and still have her in the way that they always had.

According to any book/leaflet/website you care to read about teenagers and cancer, when presented with this situation they are likely to withdraw/sulk/ignore the problem/ shoplift/start setting fire to cars. Maybe some do. Mine didn't. Mine talked, and asked questions, and came to the hospital, and looked after me, and generally behaved in a way that made me deeply proud, and at the same time sad, sad, sad that they should have to.

BAH! THINKING 🧚

What is cancer like?

Cancer is a big, scary disease. If you have a cancer, thinking of it as a big, scary disease isn't very helpful. I think it's a good idea to find a different way to think about cancer: a way that makes it less frightening, more manageable. Here are some suggestions. You might choose to use one of them, or you might find your own way of thinking about a cancer.

1. Because I thought of myself as dancing with cancer, it made sense to see cancer as a dance partner. I didn't see it as being a dashing, 'May I have this dance?', twinkle-in-the-eye, steer-you-round-the-floor-so-you-feel-as-though-you're-flying partner, though. Oh no. The cancer I was dancing with was pock-marked and clumsy, with bad breath and a grip I couldn't wriggle out of. I had no respect for this partner, and I knew that the minute the music stopped playing I would wrench myself free and walk away, without a backward glance.

2. Someone told me that they saw their cancer as being like a naughty child who didn't know they were behaving badly. This allowed her to cope with cancer without becoming frustrated or upset by it: it didn't know any better.

3. Cancer could be seen as being something small and inconsequential: a tiny shadow in a corner of an otherwise bright and healthy body.

4. Cancer might be an alien or a monster, but the cartoon sort, the sort that is printed on a child's pencil case and is monster-like but not in the least bit scary.

5. Maybe a cancer is more like a ghost that needs to be exorcised, and when it is, it will vanish into the hereafter and never be able to come back.

6. You might visualize a cancer as being like a weed that needs to be pulled out of a flowerbed: dragged out by the roots, and then the earth must be treated to make sure the weed won't grow back.

7. Cancer could be seen as a teacher: the sort of teacher that everyone at school hated but later, when you look back, you see as being one of the most influential and strong people in your early years, and the person that you learned the most from. The cancer-teacher might have a hooked nose, a hard stare and some hard lessons, but you might choose to see these lessons as things you need to learn.

THE EMAILS

I sent out the email below, topped and tailed with a bit of personal chat. (I had a lot of people to get in touch with and the information was the same for everyone.)

> I'm getting in touch with a bit of bad news, which is rubbish of me, but I wanted to let you know.
>
> I've been diagnosed with a cancer in my breast. It's stage I, which is good, but aggressive, which is not so good, but apparently not surprising – if breast cancer crops up in someone as relatively young (37 is young in this context! fab!)

as me it tends to be aggressive. The prognosis is excellent (more chance of dying crossing the road), but I do have to have an operation to remove the cancer, some lymph nodes, and a dodgy-looking few cells in the other breast. That will be in the next few weeks, then there will definitely be radiotherapy after Xmas, and a possibility of chemotherapy if the nodes look nasty.

We are all a bit shocked as there's no history of breast cancer in the family, but relieved that it has been caught early. I am planning to read a lot of books, do a lot of knitting, get a lot of sleep and watch a lot of rubbish on TV while the treatment happens. My approach is very much that this is a pain in the backside rather than the cue for an existential crisis!

Sorry to hit you with bad news by email but please be reassured that I am OK. I'll let you know my op date, etc. when I know (should be within the next three weeks I think). And please recommend books, films, anything to keep me occupied ...

Responses were generally quick, and kind. Sarah told me about her friend's mum who had just recovered. Cheryl recommended books and films and told me she was sending strength and health. Hannah offered to come wig shopping and to support the family. Rob told me how his dad had recovered from cancer 20 years previously, and had taken a mental approach similar to my own. Everyone wished me well and told me I'd get better.

HOW TO HELP: Five things not to say when you get the news

1. 'Oh, that's a shame. <pause> Have you been listening to *The Archers*?'
    If you are uncomfortable talking about cancer, just say so. Say, 'I'm really sorry, but I'm going to need some time to absorb this. Is it OK if I call you back in a day or so?'

2. 'I was reading an article that said most people have a cancer because they eat too much cheese/don't get enough sleep/take the contraceptive pill.'
    Yes, it's perfectly possible that the cancer could be construed as our own fault. There are lots of studies that establish correlation, and some causation, with the Western lifestyle. Pointing this out, though, does not help.

3. 'Oh, poor you. Poor, poor you. Oh, your poor children. Your poor, poor children.'
    Most people diagnosed with a cancer will be trying very hard to focus on the positives, even if there aren't many to focus on. Acknowledgement that this is bad news is fine. Cloying pity is not.

4. 'That's terrible. That reminds me of the time when I ...'
    It's not about you, so be careful. Sharing your experience might help, and empathy matters. But make sure you're focused on the person with a cancer and not finding a new way to process your own experience.

31

5. 'You're the third person I know who's died of breast cancer.'
    Someone really did say that to someone I know. Cancer does not automatically equal death anymore, and even if it did, talking about anyone as though they are already dead is very bad manners indeed. Don't do it.

 HOW TO HELP: Ten things to say when you get the news

1. 'What can I do to help?'
    Ask the question. Write down the answer. And do it. You could offer some help, too, but try to do so without making assumptions. So don't say, 'I'll come and do your shopping for you,' because your friend might be perfectly capable of doing his/her own shopping.

2. 'What's the best way for me to support you?'
    Many people, when faced with a medical crisis, swing into 'You are now the patient and I will proceed to look after you' mode, which is sweet but infuriating. What they can forget is that, no matter how ill you are or may become, you will still, first, be yourself. Having an adult-to-adult conversation shows that you recognize this.

3. 'How are you feeling?'
    It's OK to ask, so long as you are prepared to listen to the answer.

4. 'My mother had breast cancer ten years ago. She just ran her eighteenth marathon.'

5. 'How are <insert names of partner and/or children> doing?'

   When I was diagnosed I was more concerned about Alan, my children and my parents than I was about myself. That's not because I'm any kind of a saint. I knew that I was OK, but I didn't really know whether they were, or to what extent they were showing me how they were feeling. So when people asked about my family, it gave me an opportunity to talk about them. And I was reassured that there were people looking out for the people that I loved.

6. 'What's going to happen next?'

   The more you know, the better equipped you are to understand/support/call at the right time to see how it's all going. If you hear terms you don't understand, write them down and look them up. I was happy to explain to people how I was feeling, what the prognosis was, how my treatment was going to happen. But explaining the difference between a fine-needle biopsy and a more complicated core biopsy got a bit much after the first dozen times. That's what Wikipedia is for.

7. 'You must have a lot of people to call. May I call you tomorrow?'

   Be mindful that the person who is calling you is probably tired, shocked and frightened, and has a long list of people to call. For now, it's not about you.

8. 'Is there anyone I can call for you?'

   See 7.

9. 'I'm sure you will get through this. I remember the time when you wrestled a mountain lion to stop it from eating a koala/broke your leg getting out of a taxi in ridiculously high yet fabulous red shoes, and you coped brilliantly then.'

We're not always good at recognizing, or remembering, our strengths. More than that, when cancer dances along it's easy to recast one's entire life as nothing but picnics, holidays, beer and skittles. (Although of those four supposedly fabulous things, only the holidays really do it for me. You can certainly keep your picnics, unless it's one of those picnics that comes with a candelabra.) So a reminder of how well a person diagnosed with cancer has done under trying circumstances in the past is a really powerful way to help them. Just make sure you do it without making them feel that they have to be a superhero(ine).

10. 'I am so sorry to hear that.'
    Simple. But so powerful. And so many people swing into 'Just Do Anything' mode that they forget to say this. Please, if you do nothing else, say it.

🌱 🌱 🌱

Surgery: The search for the perfect pyjamas

BAH! THINKING

A visualization to prepare you for surgery

Get comfortable. Breathe deeply and slowly. Wait until you are calm. It doesn't matter if this takes a long time.

Now imagine a series of people. (I visualized something a bit like a reception line at a wedding, with person after person coming up to me and smiling and embracing me. This might work for you, or you may find it easier to imagine hearing people speak.)

Imagine your surgeon telling you that the operation could not have gone better.

Imagine a nurse telling you how well your wounds have healed.

Imagine the people that you love telling you how well you look.

Imagine your colleagues saying that they didn't expect to see you back at work so soon.

Imagine telling each of these people in turn that you are fully recovered.

Enjoy the feelings that come with these thoughts.

Smile. Open your eyes.

Do this every day.

GETTING READY PART 1: HOSPITAL

In the week before my surgery I went to hospital three times, and did these things:

- I had blood taken, at least twice. I forget why. Or maybe I wasn't told.

- I had another core biopsy. By now I'd got wise to these babies so I took ibuprofen and paracetamol beforehand.

- I had a wire inserted into my left breast, where the dodgy-looking cells were. If that sounds kind of dinky and discreet to you, think again. The idea was that the wire pointed the surgeon to the area to be removed, because the dodgy-looking cells weren't visible to the naked eye. Very clever. I didn't really understand why the tail of this wire, which was a metre or so long (and it really was a metre, I'm not exaggerating for tragical-comical effect) had to be coiled up and taped onto the middle of my chest. Very unpleasant, especially when I lay on my side in bed and my breasts squished themselves around the coil. I did understand why the little crocodile clip was sitting on the outside of my skin – to keep the wire in place – but I wasn't very keen on that, either.

- I had more mammograms. Lots more. Fortunately, the anaesthetic from the insertion of the guide wire hadn't worn off.

- I was tested for MRSA. If you have it, the hospitals don't let you in, which seems quite sensible, although no one ever explained what would happen if I actually did have it. (I like to think I would have had the operation in the hospital car park, but I think a course of antibiotics and a postponement would have been more likely.) The testing was both painless and spectacularly undignified. I was given a cotton wool swab and asked to rub it on the inside of my cheek. So far, so good. But then I was given another, which I was asked to rub along 'the sweaty part at the side of your groin'. (I was going to take umbrage at this but realized that, as all hospitals have a base temperature in the region of 130 degrees Fahrenheit, there was a fair chance that everyone's groin-side was glowing.) So a nurse watched as I undid my trousers and poked about a bit with the swab.

- My medical history was taken, many, many times. If I had been given a cupcake every time I said 'only a tonsillectomy' I'd have gone up two dress sizes. (It would be much easier if hospitals printed the medical history questionnaire on, say, a vest, you wrote the answers on it, and every time there were questions you could simply whip your top off and there it would be.)

- I was weighed and my blood pressure was taken.

- I had radioactive blue ink injected into my right breast, next to the nipple. Honestly, it didn't hurt a bit. In fact it was done, quite literally, before I knew it.

- I had a little cry in the Cupboard of Tears. At this stage I was still insisting on doing all of these visits on my own, and in the hour between the guide wire and the radioactive injection, I got a bit overwhelmed.

GETTING READY PART 2: ELSEWHERE

If you have had a baby, the chances are that before s/he was born you went out and bought so much toothpaste, soap, washing powder and tins of baked beans that you will still be using some of them by the time that child leaves home. I remember doing that before Ned was born: I remember feeling that I must be Completely Organized because I was going to be so tired/busy/covered in sick that I would never get to a shop again. I had a similar feeling in the run-up to surgery. I got groceries delivered. I bought, wrapped and labelled all of our Christmas presents (surgery was on 19th November). I booked a massage for the day before I went into hospital, because I thought it would be best to go into it relaxed, although I didn't have it because the masseuse was afraid that the massage would 'speed cancer round the body'. (I think she may have had a slightly inflated idea of her own skills.)

I also talked to the people I work with, to let them know what was happening when, and when I planned to be back at work, and what I knew about further stages of treatment. They were all infuriatingly laid back. They said things like, 'We can pick this up whenever you're ready,' and, 'Just let me know when you feel up to it, and we'll do it then.' I wanted a diary full of commitments, as a way, I think, of proving to myself that I was going to get through all this ... but I did, eventually, see that they were right.

I tidied up, surreptitiously, so that people didn't ask me what I was doing and I wouldn't have to explain that if I died I didn't want them to have to deal with half-empty jars of dried-out foundation and bras missing one of their underwires.

But mostly, I shopped for pyjamas. I knew that if the surgeon did find cancer in the lymph nodes, he would remove them all there and then. Which meant drains, which meant needing access to drains, which meant pyjamas that buttoned up the front. Which I didn't possess.

So, between hospital appointments, and in the long afternoons when everyone was at work/school and which I had yet to learn how to fill, I looked for pyjamas. It became a little obsession, and a good way of not thinking about the bigger, scarier stuff. The pyjamas had to be cotton, because hospitals are hot. They had to be comfortable and roomy, to accommodate dressings, drains, etc. They had to be free of teddy bears, polar bears or cartoon characters, because I'd never worn that sort of thing and I was damned if I was going to start now. (Also, I was concerned that if I needed to be assertive with anyone at any point, being decked out in Disney might undermine my position.) And – this was really important – they had to be the sort of pyjamas I might have bought even if I hadn't been going into hospital for surgery to remove a cancer.

Eventually, I found them. Cotton, red, with a white trim and sprinkled with little white stars. I still wear them. I still love them. I'm still grateful to them, for being a crucial distraction when I needed it.

When I look back, I see that what I was trying to do, really, was to make sure that the world stayed the same. I was prepared to have a cancer, if absolutely necessary, but I wasn't going to let it change anything. My world would keep on turning on the same axis. Nothing would be different. Little did I know.

de Bono's Green Hat: The need for creativity

Green Hat thinking is all about unbounded new thinking. It's the Hat for new ideas – and overcoming difficulties. It's the perfect Hat to use for thinking in the run-up to surgery, because this is the time to have plans and strategies in place. And the ways that you cope with recovery don't have to be the conventional ways of coping. Green Hat thinking says: Anything goes.

BAH! THINKING

For convalescence

Here are some of the ideas that came out of my pre-surgery Green Hat thinking. They might spark some ideas of your own.

- Line up a couple of good, uplifting books to read while you are recovering. Go back to your old book-friends, or buy or borrow the latest book by a favourite author. I learned the hard way that this is not the time to tackle hard-hitting fiction or anything with very long chapters and/or very small print.

- Stock up a little bit, but don't obsess about it. Make sure you have your own staples, be they milk and bread or rice and peas, and some of whatever you consider to be a treat.

- Think about how people are going to get the news about how surgery went. Set up a telephone tree, or simply ask some people if they will then call others on your behalf. Make an email group so you can write one email to bring everyone up to date.

- Make sure the room you are going to convalesce in, whether it's your living room or your bedroom, is clean and comfortable. If anything is annoying you – the untidy bookshelf, the corner where all of the homeless items in your house gravitate to – sort it out, or get someone to sort it out for you. The chances are that you'll be spending a lot of time in that space so you need it to be relaxing and calm. Make sure that you'll have bright light for reading, and soft light for relaxing. If you're going to be watching TV, check the batteries in the remote control.

- Make a list of people who have offered to help and what you might ask them to do. If you're not sure whether you are going to be able to do something or not, put someone on standby to step in.

- Establish what the rules of your treatment and recovery are going to be. I told everyone that I would let them know if I needed something – so they didn't need to ask or second-guess me all of the time.

- Think about how you are going to cope with everyday life after surgery. I knew that I wouldn't be able to bathe until the dressings had been removed and the wound healed; so I bought some lovely bubble bath ready for when I could get back into a bath, and some creamy shower gel to wash the bits that weren't out of bounds. I'd been told that I wouldn't be able to use an underarm deodorant while the wound from the lymph node removal healed. This was mentioned in passing by someone I saw in the pre-operative clinic, and sent me into a panic. (Scarred and smelly? I don't think so.) So I bought a crystal deodorant stone. For me, being ready for these peripheral prohibitions helped me to feel in control. I didn't see – I still don't see – why having an operation should mean losing dignity or compromising on what's important to you. Personally, I like to be clean and smell nice. I don't think that's unreasonable.

• Find some fabulous pyjamas (obviously).

THINGS NOT TO DO BEFORE SURGERY

Just the one. Do not type 'breast cancer surgery' into a search engine and spend an afternoon trawling through the discussion boards and groups that come up. If you want to know why not, find a gathering of women in their early seventies and tell them that you're pregnant. They will tell you stories that will make your brain curdle and your toenails fall off. And they'll do it, not from malice, but because at the time when they gave birth no one talked about it. They just went into the back bedroom with some string and came out three days later with a baby and a really dirty look in the direction of their husband. These women didn't have a chance to deal with often traumatic birth experiences, not really, and so they deal with it by telling you about it, in high definition.

There are a lot of women out there who have had a great deal of difficulty dealing with cancer, and who, for whatever reason, have no one to talk to about it. The internet is a good place for them to come together and share their stories and their anger and their beliefs about how badly they have been treated and how unreliable surgeons are. There may be some truth in what they say. But before going into surgery is not a good time to meet them.

There are websites and discussion groups with helpful, useful and medically sound information and advice. If you want to find out more, go to the website of a cancer charity that you know, or ask your hospital for a recommendation.

SURGERY: A LONG DAY

5:30 a.m.

I get up. I don't have breakfast, though, because it's not allowed. I drink some water and put on comfortable clothes. I've been told I will be in hospital overnight, so I'm wearing something I should be able to get back into without too many problems. I wonder once more at the metre of wire looped up out of my chest.

6 a.m.

Alan and I leave for the hospital. It's nearby, so we walk, because I'm not sure how long it will be before I'm taking a 20-minute walk again. It's a clear morning, still dark. Because it's so early and I have an overnight bag, it feels as though we are going on holiday. Walking down the road, I'm struck by how odd it is to be feeling well and yet know that I have a cancer growing in my breast.

6:30 a.m.

We arrive, as instructed, at the area for patients having surgery today. This is the first point at which reality departs from my imagined version of events. I'd imagined waiting on my own, or at least with a room full of other women looking slightly bemused at how their breasts had, as it were, turned on them. Instead I am faced with a mass of people, sitting on the rows of screwed-down chairs more commonly seen in a bus station, and it's clear that (unless there is a freakishly high rate of male breast cancer in south west London) everyone having surgery today is here. We find seats near an old man, a very sad looking couple and a woman in a brown velour tracksuit that looks as though it has been bought especially for the occasion, in the same way that pink velour tracksuits in airports do. (Well, my PJs and I could relate.) We wait. We do a crossword. And then another one.

8 a.m.

People start to be called through to the cubicles. They arrive back in the waiting room shortly afterwards, wearing hospital gowns, opaque white stockings that end just below the knee, and blue hospital flip-flops. I tell Alan I will be OK from here, and he goes to work. (I'd asked him to go to work. I hated the idea of him sitting around waiting for news, although why I thought he wouldn't be doing this at work, I have no idea. But I was glad he wasn't going to see me in the gown/stocking/flip-flop ensemble.)

8:30 a.m.

I am called through to the cubicles and given the gown and stockings. Joy has manicured and painted my fingernails and toenails, but I am given a bottle of acetone and some

44

cotton wool and told to remove the varnish. My bags are taken and labelled: we'll be reunited on the ward. I give up my glasses (my usual contact lenses being forbidden) and can now see clearly for approximately 18 inches in front of my nose.

9 a.m.

It's my turn to go to theatre; I am told, in a hushed tone, that I am 'first on the list'. A nurse walks me, the sad looking lady (still accompanied by her husband) and the woman in the brown velour tracksuit to the lifts. The brown tracksuit woman (who is now in a gown, but unmistakable) has an entourage of husband, sister and mother, all complaining loudly about something. I opt not to listen to what. I don't know whether it's the situation or the fact that I can't see very far, but I am in a funny little trance. We go down in the lift and are taken to a reception area where the others are rapidly taken off in other directions and I am asked to wait. Part of me wonders whether someone will pop out and say 'Surprise! It's not cancer! We were only having you on!' I decide that if there's a camera crew I will insist that any sight of the surgical stockings must be edited out of the final cut.

9:15 a.m.

Despite my many visits to the hospital over the last couple of weeks, I have not been asked to fill in a consent form. One of the surgery team takes me through it. I sign it, signifying that I understand that if I die or am permanently disabled or brain damaged on the operating table it's just, y'know,

45

one of those things. Then we agree which breast has the cancer and the doctor takes a pen and writes, 'This one,' on my right shoulder and draws a big arrow down toward my breast. (Modern surgery is many things. Subtle is not one of them.) I notice that the pen is an ordinary felt-tip, and this tiny detail makes me want to cry – surely there should be a special pen for writing on people who are about to have a cancer removed? Mr Mokbel, my surgeon, comes over and speaks to me. I feel a little bit starstruck and wonder how many people get to meet someone who is, in all likelihood, about to save their life.

9:30 a.m.

I meet the anaesthetist and her assistant. We talk medical history. ('Only a tonsillectomy.') The needle is in the back of my hand, some painkillers are pushed through the line, and then the anaesthetic comes, and everything goes dark. I don't even get to count backwards from 10. I'm out.

Later. Maybe 1 p.m.

I start to come round in the recovery room. In that space between knowing I am awake and being able to open my eyes, I try to work out whether there is a drain in my armpit. I can't decide. I'm fuzzy round the edges, the way that you are after a general anaesthetic. My sight is fuzzy round the edges, the way it is when your glasses are in a bag on the ward with your splendid pyjamas, and without help your sight is so poor that you couldn't recognize your own mother standing under a flashing neon arrow with 'Look! It's your mother!' picked out in big red letters above it if it were more than 3 yards away. What consciousness I have seems to be concentrated around my right breast, or rather, the edges of the recently gouged wound in it. (I'm sure the surgery team was as good as it gets. But right then, I felt gouged.) And wearing an oxygen mask is very confusing, at least if you're not a scuba diver, forensics expert, elephant impersonator or other person used to having their nose and mouth enclosed.

I know what I need to know. I call, 'Nodes? Nodes?' The nurse comes over, and checks and nudges bits of me and talks to me, but she's obviously heard my cry as 'Nurse?' and so I ask about the nodes again. If all of the lymph nodes have been removed, the cancer has spread. If they haven't, it hasn't. This piece of knowledge is so important that it's bumping at the sides of my universe. The nurse vanishes from my field of vision (by walking two steps to the end of the trolley I am lying on), but I hear the rustling of paper. She says, 'They took away all of the tumour and your lymph nodes were clear.' I feel a tear slide down the side of my face and into my ear. The nurse interprets this as pain, and gives me some morphine (or, more likely, even more morphine). Darkness again.

A little later

I come round as I hear people talking over me. The nurse is discharging me to the porter, who will take me to the ward. I gather that I have had a lot of morphine and am still quite sleepy. Off I go, woozy and tired, being wheeled through the hospital corridors.

On the ward

Here reality departs from my vision once more. In my imagination: a single room, white walls, sunlight streaming in, peace. (Perhaps I was having a multi-purpose vision in case I died.) In reality, I am wheeled into a bay with four beds. Televisions are on; there are visitors; there is talking; doors are banging; somewhere, a radio rattles away. My bed has the flimsiest, most threadbare curtains outside a 1950s orphanage as the only thing between me and a world that is too abrasive and too much. I start to cry. I ask for a bed on a side ward. The nurse tells me that there aren't any. I ask again. The nurse tells me that the side rooms are for people who are really sick, and I cry some more. (I don't think she means it unkindly, not really.) I offer, rather grandly and hysterically, to pay for a side room. Still none. The nurse goes to call Alan. I keep crying, though now it's bordering on howling. I ask if I can discharge myself. Everyone starts to look a bit panicky. My blood pressure is taken and I am ticked off because it is going up. Cathy, the Macmillan nurse that I like, is (it seems to me) shoved through the curtains by the ward nurse as my sobs soar. Cathy holds my hand. I get some words out. 'Vulnerable' is one. 'Private' is another. 'Too much' I say, over and over. Cathy nods and tells me it's OK. I tell her I want to be on my own. As I do so I realize that the ward around me has gone quiet. Either everyone's gone or everyone's listening. I think I know which. Cathy says that she can't get me a room but she can get me a key to a private garden. The ludicrousness of this – it's November, I'm hooked up to a drip; getting me to a garden would require wheelchairs, porters and getting very cold – makes me stop for long enough to get a grip and calm my breathing and start to see straight again.

Later

Alan arrives. I ask the nurse, who looks a bit less scared of me now, whether I can go home. Apparently, if I eat something, walk a little bit, and go to the loo, I can.

6 p.m.-ish

Having demonstrated my ability to keep food down, get myself to the loo and pass urine (they take my word for that part), I am discharged. I'm given an injection to stop my blood clotting, a leaflet of arm exercises and a warning that I must never have injections, blood taken or blood pressure readings in my right arm again. 'Never ever?' I ask. 'Never ever.' I'm shocked by this.

7 p.m.-ish

Louise collects us from the hospital and drives us home. I put on my pyjamas (hooray!) and get into my own bed, which feels like the best and safest place in the world. I think about how there is no cancer in my body.

8 p.m.

Ned, Joy and their dad come round. Joy has made me a penguin with a pocket on the front, which holds a note saying 'Hello Stephanie, I'm Dusk the penguin, and I'm here to keep you company. Your son and daughter love you very much, so keep going ... and please, don't give up.' I cry. There are flowers and chocolates and we talk about the day. Joy seems calm; Ned is distraught by the bruises already blooming out from behind the dressings. Joy goes back to her dad's; Ned elects to stay, but has to be persuaded to sleep in his own bed, rather than at the foot of mine. My heart breaks a little bit more. I talk to my parents. I probably eat something. Probably chocolate.

9 p.m.

Painkillers. Sleep.

AFTER

Frankly, recovering from surgery was pretty dull. I will say two things, though. The first is that people were amazingly kind. My GP dropped in on his way home from work to see how I was doing. Alan, Ned and Joy quietly kept me going, making tea, keeping me company, watching me sleep. Alan helped me to shower while making me feel that being unable to take an unaided shower was completely normal. Mum came down from Northumberland and knitted with me, and she brought gingerbread and presents from Auntie Susan, a bag of them, one to open every day for ten days.

And the second thing is this. It didn't take as long as I thought to recover.

Here is my third blog post, ever.

MONDAY, 1 DECEMBER 2008 (ABRIDGED): WHAT A DIFFERENCE A FORTNIGHT MAKES

Day 1:

I have operation and come home. I think I'm doing OK until I see the shock on the children's faces when they see me. Sleep like a baby apart from the bits where I accidentally roll onto my front.

Day 2:

The remains of the anaesthetic wells through me again and again and I nap, wake, nap, wake, nap, and sleep like a baby again. I email everyone to let them know I'm OK and somehow, this is exhausting. The flowers and cards start arriving. I cry when I open them.

Day 3:

I sit downstairs for a while and this, too, is exhausting. Knitting and watching TV help me to feel [a] ... bit more human. I can't concentrate on reading though, which is horrid, and makes me cry.

Day 4:

I get dressed! Yay. (Also exhausting, but I don't cry.)

Day 5:

I venture out into the great wide world with Alan. We walk to the café round the corner and I have a little sob when we get there, and feel as though I will never be back to normal. Alan reminds me that it's less than a week since my op and I should be patient. We both laugh at this as I was too impatient to queue for the patience when it was given out. I say positive stuff about recovery, time etc (but secretly don't mean it).

Day 6:
Alan, Ned, Joy and I go to Starbucks. I'm very excited by this as it feels like a normal thing to do. I'm so excited that I even take photos while there (which is clearly not very normal. I mean, who takes photos of themselves in Starbucks?)

Even manage a little light shopping afterwards, although it is Joy who brings me home rather than the other way round.

Day 7:
Alan goes back to work and I am collected by Lou and Ellis who look after me without making me feel as though I need looking after. I am grateful …

Day 8:
… but being properly on my own makes me realise that I do need a bit of looking after, after all. I am weepy on and off all day. I take myself to the café round the corner as a way of distracting myself, and some very dinky babies are there with their mums to remind me that actually, it's not always all about me. Mum arrives at 4.45pm and I cry when I see her.

Day 9:
Results day – and not quite as clear cut or positive as I hoped. […] Mum, Alan and I share a bottle of wine in

the evening – my first drink since the op – another sign of progress?!

Day 10:

Alan goes off to a meeting and won't be back until the next day, which I am pathetic about, then feel bad about afterwards. I have a bath!!! Yay!!!! As having a bath is my main coping strategy in life, not being able to have one has been miserable.

Make dinner for the first time (well, heat up pie and cook some vegetables) and talk to my Auntie Susan, who makes me laugh so much that I am reassured that my pelvic floor, at least, must be in good shape.

Day 11:

Mum, Joy and I go to Kingston, and I take all of it in my stride – the noise, the people, the travel (they take the mickey out of me for knitting on the bus), the shops. I get jostled a couple of times which makes me wince, but other than that I could be any old cancer-free person. Buy hats and don't cry all day.

Day 12:

Mum leaves, Alan and I potter around at home, and I realise how much I am going to miss working over the next little while. [...] I look at my diary and see that I was scheduled to train next week, and feel very sorry for myself. Give myself a chat about being able to work during bouts of chemotherapy, innovative new ways of working, etc, and feel a bit better.

Day 13:

Give myself more chats about being able to work during bouts of chemotherapy, innovative new ways of working, etc, and feel a bit better. Talk to my hairdresser about cutting off most of my hair later this week if I do need to have chemotherapy. I'd rather get rid of it when feeling relatively sane than wait until I am having mood swings and feeling rough.

Day 14:

Here I am, home alone, no tears and feeling like a normal person (albeit a normal person wearing a hat indoors so everyone can get used to it, just in case).

What a difference a fortnight makes. So maybe, day by day by day, I will get through all this.

BAH! THINKING

Recovery plan

Post-surgery is not the best time for just letting things happen. Days are long, your body is confused and nothing is quite as it should be. So it's a good idea to think and plan some ways of coping. Here are some of the things I did.

1. Drink a lot of water. It helps flush all of the anaesthetic out of your system. And then you have to go to the loo, which means you have to get up and move, which is good, too.

2. Plan your day. When you don't have a lot of energy, or when you're in pain, a day can seem like a long, long time. So even if your plan is, 'I'll read for an hour this morning,

then I'll have a sleep, then I'll get up for lunch, then I'll knit until *Deal or No Deal* is on,' you've given yourself some structure.

3. If you're allowed to, try to move. Try to breathe some different air. Try to keep your world just a little bit bigger than your bedroom.

4. If anything you're unsure about happens, write it down, and ask someone (for preference, a qualified medical professional rather than Dr Google.) This is not a time to be self-effacing or take a 'wait and see' approach.

5. If you have drugs, write down what you take and when you take it. When all of your days are a bit samey, it can be difficult to remember when the last lot of paracetamol was.

6. Don't be afraid to ask for what you want. It might be company, or it might be peace. For me, it was important that I was left on my own for a while, just so I could see for myself that I could cope and that I wasn't becoming an invalid. The people around you want to support you, but you might have to tell them how.

7. Don't look too far ahead. If you do what your body needs to do today, tomorrow will be easier. That's all you need to worry about, for now.

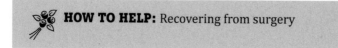 **HOW TO HELP:** Recovering from surgery

1. Recognize and support all of the above.

2. Before surgery happens, sit down and have a conversation about what the person having surgery thinks they might need afterwards. You're not trying to tie them down to

anything, and they might not know. But they might have some ideas. (Be prepared for those ideas to change later.)

3. Try to be pro-active in your approach. I knew that my family would get/make/go out and buy anything I wanted to eat or drink, for example, but being able to have anything at all is quite difficult, especially when your body is dealing with a trauma. So a question like, 'Would you like some tea, or some apple juice?' would often make me say, 'Ooh, yes, tea please,' while my response to, 'Would you like anything?' was more likely to be, 'No, I'm fine, thanks.'

4. Have easy, quick things to do to hand. It's difficult to bridge the gap between becoming bored and not having the concentration to do anything much. Obviously, knitting is the perfect answer to this, because an afternoon goes by really quickly one stitch at a time, but if your loved one doesn't knit, then you need other boredom-breakers. A pack of cards, today's newspaper, yesterday's crossword, an audio book ... All of these things can help a long afternoon to pass.

5. Listen. Listen to what your loved one is telling you, and listen for when they go quiet. (Don't be afraid to be quiet too.)

6. Don't feel you need to have all the answers, and don't feel that your job is to Make Them Feel Better. Post-surgery there's a good chance that your loved one will need to feel how they feel, rather than be jollied along. I'm not saying that there isn't a place for comfort, or a funny story, or trying to raise a smile. Of course there is. But the other side of cancer surgery is a bleak and uneven landscape sometimes, and survivors need the chance to get to know it.

7. Remember that the person you love is still there, and that surgery has not diminished them, and that cancer does not define them. Behave accordingly.

4

Keeping a record: Better out than in

BEARING UP

There are many things that made my dance with cancer bearable. Most of those things are people: family, friends, compassionate health practitioners (lovely), inconsiderate health practitioners (the outrage powered me for days).

But, people aside, I think the major sustaining factor through what I now admit was the most difficult year of my life was my blog.

I don't think I could bear to admit it was difficult at the time. I was afraid, I think, of what might happen if I did. I was afraid that I would take up residence under the duvet and never really come out again. Maybe I was even afraid that if I admitted how Big and Challenging and Scary cancer was, I would be more likely to die of it. I don't know. All I know is that the difficulty hovered nearby, and I knew it was there, but I wouldn't engage with it. A bit like being at the same wedding as the ex-boyfriend you never quite got over: you don't speak to him, but you know where he is every second. So through most of my dance with cancer I was blithely telling everyone it was 'fine, really fine, honestly no big deal, really absolutely not as bad as I thought it would be', and this was mostly true, but a little bit not.

de Bono and Concept Extraction

Concept Extraction is a Lateral Thinking™ tool to help to find alternative ways of doing something. Let's say, for example, that you want to cheer yourself up: the obvious idea might be to go on holiday. Concept Extraction suggests that, rather than heading straight for the travel agent, you should ask yourself: what is the concept in going on holiday that makes it a good way of achieving my goal of cheering myself up? The answer could be that being in new surroundings is what's attractive. So the next question to ask is: how else could I achieve the feeling of being in new surroundings? Well ... I could take a little trip to visit a friend. I could go to a place nearby that I've never been to before but always meant to. I could paint my living room. I could ask to work out of a different office for a while. I could look for a secondment at work. I could invite a friend to stay with me and that will give me a fresh perspective on my life. And so on. Concept Extraction multiplies your ideas. And it's a great tool for helping to make a change in something that's not quite working.

One Sunday, shortly after surgery, I was ploughing through emails from people who were wishing me well and wanting to know how I was doing. I was boosted by the fact that so many people were making such an effort, but at the same time I found the process tiring. So I did a quick Concept Extraction: what's the concept here? Well, the concept of sending all of these emails is to let a lot of people know how I am doing. How else could I achieve that? I could send out more frequent group emails, I could arrange teleconferences, I could post or email a weekly round-robin, I could delegate my email-answering to Alan, Ned and Joy. I could start a blog.

I COULD START A BLOG

On 29 November 2008, I put fingers to keyboard and started the Bah! to cancer blog. I chronicled my appointments, my treatments, my feelings. I photographed and posted the hair loss and the scarring. I wrote about the people and the activities that kept me going. I was pleased and excited that people were reading it; but what mattered was what the blog allowed me to do. Because I didn't want to write one of those 'I got up. I had a shower. I felt tired and went back to bed LOL' blogs, I tried to find insights and analyse my experience. I tried to explain and expand my positive, mind-centred approach to my dance with cancer. And in doing that, I processed my experience. Before I wrote, I had to understand what I was writing about. So every day, as I wrote a blog post, I sorted something out in my mind. And that, I think, has been more important than anything else in terms of getting through a dance with cancer relatively emotionally and psychologically intact.

THURSDAY, 11 DECEMBER 2008 [ABRIDGED]: ON BLOGGING

I think I owe an apology to bloggers, and their readers, everywhere.

Until I started this blog, I had a fairly low opinion of the genre. Maybe I'd been unlucky in some of the ones I'd looked at, but so many of them seemed to go like this:

"Pies!

Today I was hungry so I thought I'd have a pie. Here's a picture of the pie. Here's a picture of me eating the pie. Here's a picture of me after eating the pie. Yum!"

To then be followed by 422 comments along the lines of "Looks like a nice pie!" and "What kind of pie was it?" and "Maybe I should have a pie … what does everyone else think?"

Now I like a pie as much as the next woman (probably more, unless the next woman is my friend Lou) but the blog thing seemed like a phenomenal waste of time.

How wrong I was. For 3 reasons:

1. I've found the process of writing the blog calming and healing

2. Many, many people have offered me support and emailed me with useful stories and tips as a result of the blog

3. I've had a browse around […] and found plenty of intelligent, insightful and entertaining blogs.

So… sorry, bloggers and blog readers. (I think I might start a pie blog next.)

BAH! THINKING

Processing your experience

There are more ways than one of processing your experience. Here are some suggestions. I don't think it matters how you do it; the key is to do it every day or so, so you're dealing with cancer a little chunk at a time. You might choose to look back over this record later; you might never revisit it. It doesn't matter.

1. Start a blog. It's dead easy. It's free, if you have internet access. There are no blog police checking your spelling and grammar.

2. Keep a diary, and make a quiet time of day to write in it. (If you are being treated for a cancer, chances are you will have plenty of times to choose from.)

3. Buy a blank notebook and draw a picture that represents your feelings in it every day.

4. Take a photograph of yourself every day, and name the photograph with a couple of words that sum up how you feel that day.

5. Ask someone to listen to you, without interrupting, for five minutes per day as you tell them how you are feeling and what's happening.

6. Sit quietly for five minutes a day. Ask yourself the question, 'What's happening?' and let your thoughts wander. You might want to have a notebook to hand to write down what comes out of these minutes – it can be surprising.

BAH! THINKING 🐉

A visualization for figuring out what's going on

Get comfortable. Make sure you are warm. When you are ready, close your eyes.

Imagine that you are walking down a corridor. On either side of the corridor are a series of closed doors. All of the doors are different. Some are ornately carved in ash and oak; some are metal; there's a barn door, a glass door, a beaded curtain.

One of these doors is the door into how you feel today. You'll know it when you see it.

When you see it, open the door and walk into the cool, light room beyond. Maybe your shoes make a noise on the floor. Maybe you are barefoot. Maybe the room is carpeted.

Somewhere in the room is something that tells you what's important to you today. It might be a word written on a piece of paper on the windowsill. It might be a painting on the wall, a piece of graffiti, a sculpture. Whatever it is, it will be immediately clear to you what it is communicating. Look at it. Think about it. Get comfortable with it.

Now, check around the room to see if there is another door. If there is, go through it to see what there is in the other room – what there is behind the feeling in the first room.

When you have learned what you need to learn today, open your eyes.

If you want to, write down what you have found.

🌱 🌱 🌱

5

I don't think so: On being a patient

DISCLAIMER

So, here's the thing. The National Health Service is brilliant, because it saved my life, because when the lump turned out to be the cancer my feet barely touched the ground, because I have had the best medical treatment that money can buy, without any direct cost to me. (You should see my holiday insurance premiums, but we can't blame Beveridge for that.) I know this. I appreciate this. I will pay my tax bills with a minimum of grumbling forever because of this.

I know that private medicine exists and I know that many people choose to take advantage of it and that's entirely up to them. I have no issue with that at all. But for me, a health service that is free at the point of need is something to be proud of, something to be supported: and I am proud to have supported it by allowing it to poke my breasts, stick many different needles into me and pump me full of nastiness. Go NHS!

Please, take this as read, and read on. It doesn't make what I'm about to say any less true.

MONDAY, 23 MARCH 2009 [ABRIDGED]:
... AND THERE'S BAD.

My meeting with the oncologist was, to put it mildly, less than satisfactory.

I've published the questions below [...] and given the answers underneath. Anything in " " is a direct quote, otherwise I'm giving you the gist. If it all reads pretty curtly ... that's a fair representation. My additional comments are in italics.

Why am I so breathless if there's nothing disastrously wrong with my lungs/heart/blood count?

Don't know. It's just a side effect. *(She did later listen to my lungs and heart and suggest I go for an echocardiogram. We also agreed that although the breathlessness is not great, it's not getting any worse, and I am managing it better. This part of the consultation was fine.)*

Is there anything we can do about my swollen feet, ankles and hands?

"Not really. It's the chemo."

Note: my hands are so swollen that my normally slightly loose engagement ring won't come off, and my legs go more or less in a straight line from foot to calf, smothering where my ankles used to be. I couldn't even wear my pirate boots at the weekend, as they wouldn't fasten over my ankles... sniff

Note 2: I went to Boots afterwards and bought an over-the-counter diuretic. So there was something that could be done.

I had a terrible taste in my mouth for about a week after the last round of chemotherapy – this is new, and so are the sleeping tablets. Which is it likely to be?

"Don't know. It could be either."

The sinus pain which begins as soon as the third chemotherapy drug is administered seems to go on longer and longer each time. Why?

After checking which of the drugs it was, "You could ask the nurses on the chemotherapy unit."

The heartburn is getting worse. Is this normal?

If the heartburn is getting worse stop taking the anti-inflammatories. You could try Gaviscon. The drug you're taking (Omeprazole) is the strongest one we have.

Note: I'm not sure whether Omeprazole is the strongest but I think there are variants available.

What is the reason for the tiredness?

It's a side effect.

Do the hot flushes mean an early menopause, or are they just hot flushes?

Could be either. You may find that your periods stop and then start again. Don't assume you're not fertile.

Once the chemotherapy is over, how soon will the side effects disappear?

I forgot to ask this. I was losing the will to live at this point. My dragon was breathing down my neck to keep me going. [I'll be introducing you to my dragon soon.]

What about the aches and pains?

"It's a side effect. You are having chemotherapy. You're nearly at the end now."

I asked about painkillers and was told to take paracetamol, despite having given a fairly detailed account of (what I consider to be) the unacceptable level of pain I'm in for much of the time. My dragon poked me with her claw. I questioned whether paracetamol was the best course of action. The oncologist said,

"There isn't a magic pill."

This may be the case, but there are several other painkillers/ drugs with a painkilling side effect that are listed on cancer help websites as options. I'm no pharmacist, but even I know that there is more to pain relief than ibuprofen and paracetamol.

Is there any reason why I can't do some nice, quiet, one to one yoga classes during my treatment?

"No, you can do anything you like, really."

Note: that reads badly in view of the previous responses, but I think it was meant kindly, as in 'don't let chemotherapy get in the way of you leading your life.'

I don't think the anti-emetics I am taking agree with me – they make me feel jittery and headachey. Can we try something else?

I didn't bother asking this: I had a funny feeling that I knew what the response was going to be. Even my dragon was rolling her eyes and sighing, in a 'let's stop wasting our time here' sort of a way.

Grrrr.

There are three things that I am annoyed about here. No, four.

1. Before my first chemotherapy session, the SHO/oncologist I saw told me that under no circumstances was I to suffer in silence, because there were plenty of drugs and plenty of ways to help me with the side effects of chemotherapy.

2. I may not be the most interesting chemotherapy candidate: I'm not fighting for my life or having unpredictable side effects, and I can still walk and talk. But that doesn't make my own experience of chemotherapy less real, or my pain and discomfort any less valid. Yes, I'm doing relatively well. But I don't think that means I should get the brush off.

3. Without exception, everyone else I have dealt with so far has been kind and involved and interested. They have done their best to make this dance as easy on me as it can possible be. It's such a shame that a senior person should be letting the side down.

4. Although I may be nearly done with chemotherapy, if we assume that side effects last for three weeks, I have 6 weeks of dealing with fairly chronic heartburn, joint pain, tiredness, and breathlessness ahead. I don't think it's unreasonable to ask for a bit of help, and to be given it.

It's interesting to get another perspective, and I was fortunate that Joy was with me. She says, "It was her [the oncologist's] job and she was getting paid for it and she just wasn't bothering at all. She was very rude and disrespectful and she seemed to think she knew best when she'd never experienced it. Everyone else was very nice, and seemed to acknowledge that I was there too." I got brusqueness rather than rudeness, but it's fair to say that I wasn't feeling especially respected.

(My dragon is feeling a little subdued. Perhaps the fact that we were at St George's hospital took it out of her, too.)

Sooo.... I will talk to the doctor on duty at the chemotherapy unit on Wednesday (with luck, it will be lovely Dr Laura, who I saw last time), and work on my visualisations, and keep my eye on all of the positives. I'm so glad that I had this extremely dispiriting consultation – and these side effects – so late on in the dance with chemotherapy. Three weeks on Thursday, the treatments will all be over. Hallelujah.

MY HOSPITAL HYPOTHESIS

There are more sick people than there are hospital places. There are more sick people than there are appointment times. There are more tests than there is time to do the tests in. There are more samples than the path labs can easily process. There are, very often, more people than there are chairs, and beds. There are not enough cleaners. There is not enough natural light. All of these things – except maybe the light, which is down to poor architecture – come down to one thing, pretty much: there is not enough money.

Because there is not enough money, the entire NHS is built on an elaborate structure of interlocking queues that make no sense. If you drew it, it would look like something by Escher, but on a day when Escher had a hangover and a deadline and, frankly, couldn't care less.

How seriously ill you are dictates your maximum queuing time, which does make a sort of sense. So, I had to have my operation within 28 days of diagnosis. I had to start herceptin within three months of finishing chemotherapy. What's good for me as a patient often translates into a target for the hospital like this, which is fair enough, as the hospital then has a clear incentive for getting treatment sorted. This usually works ... sort of.

Queues feed into other queues, and that sometimes works and sometimes doesn't. I needed to have an additional scan and core biopsy between diagnosis and surgery, but the waiting lists at the scanning department (whose queue lengths are allowed to be longer) meant that the only appointment they could offer me was three weeks *after* my operation. Each area of the hospital operates its own queueing system, so if you are being treated by oncology, you are in their recurring queue, but you then have to go for blood tests (Phlebotomy, which favours the 'take a ticket and wait' queueing system) and heart checks (Cardiac Investigations), the results of which can have an impact on your place in the oncology queue.

It's all very complicated. But that's just the background: the impact, I think, is the critical thing. For the people who work in the NHS, I imagine that all they see is an endless queue of people heading their way. I imagine that, at the beginning, they make an effort to treat every patient as unique. I imagine that, as time goes on – and mindful of the queue ever-growing in the clinic outside, and on the waiting lists beyond – patients start to blend into one, and illnesses start to fall into broader and broader categories. I imagine it becomes more about numbers, and targets, and easy, quick, default decisions, than it does about people.

I imagine that, in this scenario, there's a dream patient. The dream patient:

- does as s/he is told
- doesn't ask too many questions
- doesn't complain
- is a little bit scared of doctors and even more scared of dying
- waits as long as necessary in clinics, in queues, in waiting rooms.

I completely understand why that patient is, well, so darned dreamy. That patient is not me.

de Bono's Blue Hat

The Blue Hat is the Hat for process control. So while the other five hats are thinking about the topic, the Blue Hat is thinking about the thinking: checking that everything being offered under White Hat is information, making sure that Red Hat isn't justified or explained, encouraging Green Hat thinking to be without judgement, and so on. The Blue Hat wearer will also have a clear idea of where the thinking needs to be going. Typically, a group of people using the Six Thinking Hats® will appoint someone to wear the Blue Hat, but any of them can put the Blue Hat on themselves if they feel that the direction of the discussion needs to be looked at.

The Blue Hat helps to keep thinking on track. It allows thinking to be effective and to meet the current need. And even if you are thinking on your own, you can still use the Blue Hat to check that you are thinking usefully.

Away from a hospital, I am someone who is fairly confident, pretty assertive, and behaves well. I behave well in my personal life: I'm no paragon, but I try to be respectful, and listen, and be kind and understanding and accommodating. I behave well in my professional life: I do what I say I am going to do, when I say I am going to do it, I'm polite, I'm prompt, and I know what I'm talking about. If I see a problem, I do my best to solve it. If I need help, I ask for it. I'm lucky enough to live a life where most of the people I live and work with behave well, too. The Blue Hat plays a big role in my life. At work I am often wearing it. In my own thinking, I am used to process and clarity and goals.

People like me don't fit well into the NHS queueing system. When I was first diagnosed with a breast cancer I think I assumed that hospitals would operate like other areas of my life: I would be part of the process, and I would have a role in my treatment and recovery (apart from staying still while people stuck needles into me). I wasn't about to become a cancer expert but I was an expert in me, and surely, I reasoned, what I knew about me would be important?

Reading that last sentence over, I'm struck by how arrogant it sounds. But it's not meant to be, and I don't think it was at the time, either. (It was more to do with the idea that I had important White Hat thinking to contribute.) I was never in any doubt that there were people in much greater need of treatment than I was: the briefest of glances around the queue of waiting rooms I sat in told me that. And I was quite prepared to do as I was told: I didn't think I knew better than the medics. I didn't expect the NHS to heave its great bulk around a new centrepoint, Stephanie-who-never-for-a-moment-thought-she-would-get-a-cancer.

Here are some other things, though, that I didn't expect:

- I didn't expect to be left in a waiting room for anything up to 2½ hours with no explanation. If someone had explained things to me, fine. But – in breast clinics and oncology clinics in particular – the waits went on, and on, and on, and there never seemed to be any attempt to improve things. Waiting was simply accepted. So much so that there is a board in some clinic areas with a section marked 'waiting times', and there are laminated pieces of card that the receptionist can stick to the board, one of which says '90 minutes'. Someone has printed and laminated, in effect, the fact that it's appropriate for scared, anxious, unwell people to wait for an hour and a half. I really didn't expect that.

- I didn't expect clinics which do the same thing over and over again to be disorganized. For example, every time I went to clinic during chemotherapy, my blood pressure would be checked. I would be called into the consulting room, then the nurse would go to find a blood-pressure monitor, which could take anything up to 10 minutes. Every time. No one ever thought to get a blood-pressure monitor and leave it in the room where the patients were seen.

- I didn't expect there to be such a clear divide between side effects that mattered and side effects that didn't. The side effects that mattered tended to be anything that affected the heart – most cancer drugs don't do a lot for the cardiac muscle and it needs to be closely watched – and anything that would stop treatment from continuing. Anything else, no matter how uncomfortable or difficult, was blithely dismissed. Although this seems fairly sensible on the uber-practical 'so many patients, so little time' level, on the experiential level, it's crap. I spent a day having my heart and lungs tested because I reported the slightest of flutterings in my chest: I sat in a chair, crying and crying because I ached so much, while the next round of chemotherapy (likely to make the pain worse) was pumped into me.

• I didn't expect that my decision to work as much as I was able would be considered to be 'not taking my treatment seriously'. This was said to my face only once, but I very often found that when I did bring up questions about side effects, the topic of work did sidle in.

Me: 'I have terrible diarrhoea.'

Oncologist: 'Hmm. Yes. You're working, aren't you?'

Me: 'Yes, but as my job does not involve eating peaches and prunes all day, I fail to see how that is relevant.' (I didn't actually say that. But in a parallel universe I did, and in that universe the oncologist was so chastened that she not only apologized to me but booked herself on a month-long course in 'Communication, Empathy and Why the Person Who Can Tell How Much Pain They Are In Is, In Fact, the Patient, and Not You. Beginner level.')

• I didn't expect to be treated as anything less than an intelligent individual engaged in her own recovery. Sometimes this happened. Sometimes it didn't.

BAH! THINKING

Keeping control

Once I'd realized that I wasn't going to get the Most Favourite Most Perfect Patient (Oncology) Award 2009, I decided that I'd go for Glad To See The Back Of Her 2009 instead. (There wasn't an actual prize associated with that one. Just a big sigh of relief from both sides.) I wasn't unpleasant, or unkind, or unreasonable. But I did take steps to make sure I was getting the information and medical treatment that was best for me. I did a lot of Blue Hat thinking and tried to create process and control where there wasn't any. If this sounds like something you need to do, think about these:

1. Ask lots of questions. Write them down before you go in to see people. Then write down the answers. I went into meetings and got out my notebook and pen, and the person I was seeing would sit up straighter and pay more attention instantly.

2. Leave telephone messages that say what you want to happen and what you will do if it doesn't: something like, 'I'd really appreciate it if someone could call me back today, which is Thursday, or by noon tomorrow at the latest. If I haven't heard by then I'll call again.'

3. See if you can figure out the formula your hospital uses for email addresses. Once you have one email address you can usually extrapolate, so if your caseworker gives you the email address katy.roberts@hospital.gov.uk then you can probably safely assume that the formula is firstname. lastname@hospital.gov.uk. This means that you can email

anyone you need to with questions or concerns that you have – and you can create an email trail of your responses. Bear in mind, though, that you are not the only patient, and save this approach for anything complicated or unusual. I emailed the Sister of the chemotherapy unit when I was having problems with a tooth and didn't know what treatment I could or couldn't have before it was sorted out, and no one else seemed able to tell me. I had to go through what the dentist, the GP, the oncologist said, and give some important bits of my dental history (crucially: 'fights like devil when sedated'). Writing it all down and sending it off was easier and quicker for both the nurse and me.

4. Be clear about what's important to you. It was always really important to me that I worked; but, if I wasn't working, I didn't really care when my appointments were. It could be that you're not working but you do like to be at home in time for when the children get back from school, or that you always keep your Tuesdays free because that's when you see your group of friends. If you are clear about what matters to you then your hospital team should be able to help – so long as you are reasonable. I don't think there's anything wrong with asking for treatment to be avoided on every other Thursday. If you're only free every fifth Thursday, though, you might run into problems.

5. When someone tells you that something needs to happen – that you will be sent an appointment, or called in for a test, or have your drug regime reviewed, ask questions like, 'When will I hear from you about that?' and note the answer in your diary, and then ask, 'Who should I contact if it hasn't happened by then?' and write that down, too. Then, if you don't get that appointment, make that call.

Appointments do get not-made, letters not-sent, in a hospital dealing with thousands of patients. If you chase yours, courteously but firmly, then maybe the person who has to re-issue it will remember how courteous (and firm) you were next time, and make sure that letter goes in the postbag rather than just in that approximate direction.

6. Always find out what your appointments are for. Before I started the ALLTO drug trial (more about this in Chapter 11), I was sent an appointment for the oncology clinic. I waited a record-breaking (for me; you may have done better) 2 hours and 45 minutes. When I was eventually seen, I was asked to sign a consent form, which took all of 30 seconds. (It was the usual 'I understand that if any of the nasty things listed below happen to me or if I die it will certainly not be the hospital's fault' form and I wouldn't have been treated without signing it.) If I'd known the appointment was just for that, I'd have arranged to sign the form when I went in to collect the trial drugs the next day. Your hospital is unlikely to join dots up for you. You need to do that part yourself.

7. Accept that some things you don't like are going to have to happen and these are not the fault of the person who is treating you. There is no point in blaming the oncologist for the fact that your hair is falling out, or getting annoyed with the nurse who can't get a needle into a vein because all accessible veins are collapsing under the stress of treatment. Under these circumstances, be gracious, kind and generous, and accept that you are all doing your best in a set of trying and undesirable circumstances. (I think a good default position is to be gracious, kind and generous whenever you can anyway. You should see how many 'only £2 per month' direct debits to charities I've got going on, though.) Which brings me to ...

8. Be nice. 'Two things cost nothing,' my grandma used to say, 'Manners and a smile.' Even if you can't quite do the second some days, try for the first. I cringe when I hear people being rude ... and, in the interests of full disclosure, I must say I cringe when I remember telling a nurse that 'I do have a life, you know.' She had just rather high-handedly moved my chemotherapy back by a week because there was a bank holiday; I'd told her that I couldn't do the next week because I was working away; she'd told me I 'should be more flexible'. So, it wasn't unprovoked. But I do regret it.

9. Remember that there is such a thing as an emergency. People do need to get ahead of you sometimes. Usually those people are a shade of pallid that you never want to be, and their need is clear. Use that extra time you've just gained to remember that, however bad it is, at least you are not a scant two skin tones away from the hereafter.

MONDAY, 14 DECEMBER 2009 [ABRIDGED]: A TALE OF TWO CLINICS

Yesterday morning, I had an appointment to see the oncologist. (I no longer say 'my oncologist' for the same reasons I have never said 'my cancer': I'm not taking ownership of something that doesn't do me any good.) My appointment was at 9am, and I arrived at 9am, to a clinic waiting area already crammed with people. (There were two other clinics – Spinal Clinic and AAP Clinic, whatever that may be – going on in the same space.) Even though I was the first person to be seen and had the first appointment, it was 9.20am before I was shown into a consulting room, and 9.30am before I saw anyone. 'Twas ever thus…. but I dread to think how long the people with the last appointment at 12.30 had to wait. They are probably still there now. I hope they brought sandwiches. (And knitting.)

Anyway. I saw an oncologist (or registrar, or senior house officer) I'd not met before. This is always a little cause for hope in my foolish breast(s) but it was clear pretty much straight away that the 'hooray! some support and interest from the oncology department!' bunting could stay in the box in the loft:

Oncologist: So. You're three quarters of the way through your herceptin!

Me: I thought I was having herceptin for a year?

Oncologist: (flicking through notes) Yes, I should think so.

Me: So that will be 18 treatments?

Oncologist: Something like that, yes.

Me: I've had 7.

Oncologist: OK, so you're half way.

Me: (doggedly) Well, just over a third.

I'm sorry, but as I'm trying very hard to be realistic and not round things up, I don't see that other people should be allowed to do it on my behalf. And the last time I looked, 7 was three quarters of nine and a third, and half of fourteen. Hmph.

Anyway. we had the *Last Period Conversation* that we always have, and I talked about my tooth – let's just say that I'm glad I wasn't holding out any hope for help with that – and then there was the question of an echocardiogram. This is an ultrasound scan of the heart to check that all is well, and it needs to be done every 3 months when you are on herceptin. Apparently I'd been due one on 4 December, but I didn't get the appointment so we needed to arrange another one. (I'm writing this as though it all happened in one conversation, with one person, but actually there was so much coming and going that it was like a French farce, only without the sex and the laughs. And the vicars.)

So. As the oncologist was done with me I waited while someone else tried to re-arrange my echocardiogram appointment. I stood in the waiting area, and the person on the phone talked to me from the desk where she was on hold, over the queue of at least 6 people waiting to be checked in. All the time, the oncologist, registrar, Macmillan nurse, and two drug trial nurses were coming and going, interrupting each other, trying to sort out several things at once.... while the oncology patients waited, grey-faced and resigned, for their turn. I offered to go to the Cardiac Investigations Unit on my way out and make my own appointment. This was greeted with some consternation – why didn't I wait 10 minutes and then they would call again – but I took a deep breath, put on my snowball hat, and turned my back on oncology clinic for another 3 months. I really couldn't stand it any more.

When I got to Cardiac Investigations – which is in the new wing of the hospital, so is bright and fairly spacious and lacks the underground-bunker quality of Oncology –

I explained the situation to Pamela, the receptionist, who asked me to take a seat while she found my record. I did. After less than 5 minutes, she came out from behind the desk, came over to me, and asked whether I would like to have the echocardiogram now, to save me another trip to the hospital. I said that I would, and I was called by Katerina before another 5 minutes had passed. She knew why I was there, and she did the echocardiogram, and afterwards she showed me the screen with the results on, and I saw a picture of my heart, chugging blood through ventricles without a care.

[...]

Here are the things that Cardiac Investigations did that Oncology could do:

go up to patients and talk to them, rather than calling across rooms/desks/waiting areas

look at the notes before seeing the patient

treat the patient as an individual and a person rather than a walking disease

have one conversation at a time

keep conversations between staff about patients to a minimum in public areas

have a system for seeing patients that works.

And here are some additional tips for Oncology, just out of the kindness of my still-beating heart:

if the first appointment is at 9am, either arrive at 8.30am to prepare, or have the first appointment at 9.30am

if you keep someone waiting, let them know how long they will be waiting, and apologise – don't assume they have nothing to do but sit around while you scurry about

get organised with everything you need – file, data, appointment history, blood pressure monitor – before seeing a patient

remember that the people you are dealing with may be scared, and tired, and probably see this appointment as an important part of their recovery, and treat them accordingly

remember that just because it doesn't interfere with treatment, doesn't make it unimportant

and – I know I said this two minutes ago but I think it bears repeating – at a bare minimum, have the respect for your patient to READ THE NOTES. Or, just don't bother with the notes and have the same conversation every time. One or the other. I truly don't mind which. But don't walk into my appointment carrying my file and then immediately demonstrate that you haven't so much as opened it.

I'm willing to admit that because of the nature of the work that I do – working with teams and organisations to help them to be better, stronger, more efficient, more focused, led more dynamically – I may be more prone to being annoyed by these things than the average cancer bunny. But even so…. I don't think this kind of service is on, really. Do you?

HOW TO HELP: Some things you can do for the patient in your life

1. Go to appointments with them. Even if they say they'll be fine. Even if they insist. Insist you know better. I always felt as though I should be able to cope with appointments on my own, as it seemed a waste of two people's mornings to sit in a waiting room. But when I got that people wanted to come along, I felt so much more comfortable.

2. Find out what's important to your loved one and agree with them beforehand what you will do to help them with it. I wish I'd asked someone to come along and help me to get proper help with chemotherapy-related stomach problems. I didn't think to ask. But I know that many of my friends would have willingly staged a sit-in in the oncologist's office until we got real answers to my questions.

3. Recognize that your loved one might be using so much energy on their dance with cancer that they might not be what you would normally expect. Be sensitive.

4. Take stuff to do to appointments. You might wait hours, and your loved one might not want to chat for hours. Also, being in a room full of sad, wasting-away people can make social chat feel tricky and inappropriate.

5. Keep a record of your loved one's regular appointments and offer to come along, rather than waiting to be asked.

6. Write down what happens when, if your loved one isn't writing things down.

7. If you are going along to anything that your loved one might find distressing – if they don't like needles and are having blood taken, for example – save a conversational distraction for the crucial moment. Gerri asked me what I was knitting while there was some very complicated line/ arm/blood stuff going on, and it really helped.

8. If you go to a meeting with an oncologist, radiotherapist, etc. with your loved one, make a point of shaking their hand and introducing yourself. They'll know you're not just there to hold the coats.

9. Afterwards, tell your loved one how well they did.

6

Chemotherapy: Enter the dragon

DECIDING

Chemotherapy wasn't in my plan. It wasn't in my surgeon's plan, either, to start with. His view was that if a 1.5-cm tumour could be removed in its entirety, and if the slightly-iffy-looking cells on my left breast were just iffy-looking and not a cancer, and if my lymph nodes were clear, showing that the cancer was not yet spreading around my body, there would be no need for chemotherapy. One of the things that kept me going through preparation for surgery and recovery was the constant thought that 'just this and a little bit of radiotherapy and some drugs and we'll be done.' I knew what a lucky girl I was. Managing to have cancer but without the chemo! I felt charmed. And I believed that the three 'ifs' would all go my way. After surgery, it looked as though I was right.

A week after the operation, and Mum and I were back at the hospital, for the Official Results and the dressing removal. We were told by one of my surgeon's registrars that:

- the tumour had been removed in its entirety,

- the iffy-looking cells in the left breast were not a problem (now I come to think of it, no one ever told me what they were, and I didn't ask – I suppose as long as they weren't another cancer, I didn't much care, and neither did anyone else),

- and the lymph nodes were clear,

- and so chemotherapy was the next thing.

Time skidded and lurched, the way a cartoon bear might when it sees a sign to a picnic area. Suddenly everything seemed very surreal. The fact that the registrar was oddly dressed didn't help. She looked as though she was going to *The Rocky Horror Picture Show* later and had laddered her tights and put on a frighteningly short skirt in preparation, so she only needed to whip her top off and put some eyeliner on and she's be ready to do the 'Time Warp' with the best of them. I know details like that shouldn't matter, but they do, they do, they do. When I questioned the need for chemotherapy – going through what my surgeon had told me – she looked a bit confused and squinted at my notes in case she'd misread them. I was searching through my mind for a word that looked like 'chemotherapy' that she could have misread it for. I didn't come up with anything, or anything that made me feel any better – if there is such a thing as crenotherapy I wasn't aware of it in an oncology context.

Panicking under the steely glare of my mother and the fact that I was clearly about to burst into tears, the registrar called in the Macmillan nurse on duty, and I was ushered into the Cupboard of Tears. Suddenly we were in the thick of a conversation about exhaustion and having your teeth checked and being sick, and being handed leaflets about ways to tie a scarf round your head in order to conceal hair loss. (To be frank, having 'baldy cancer girl' tattooed on my forehead would have done less to give the game away.)

We were told to come back and see the oncologist in a week. (Just a note, NHS: Asking someone to wait a week between being told they need chemotherapy and seeing an oncologist is not a great move.)

That week was not a good time. First of all, I don't like not knowing stuff. By which I mean, I know that most people aren't members of The Uncertainty Fan Club, but I *really* don't like not knowing things, to the extent that I would rather make a bad decision today and have A Plan, than wait until tomorrow being unsure, even if that means I could then have A Better Plan. Secondly, I was keen to get on with my life, including work, and I couldn't book anything in until I knew what my diary was going to look like. And thirdly, being told you need chemotherapy but having no additional information – how long for? what will it do to me? what will happen? – is not a good state of affairs.

Still, the week passed, as bad weeks as well as good weeks do, and Alan and I headed back to the hospital, and we met the oncologist for the first time. Although later – as you already know from the previous chapter – I developed a healthy dislike for her, on this occasion she couldn't have been more helpful.

de Bono's Yellow Hat and Black Hat

Yellow Hat thinking asks that we look at the logical benefits of something. Black Hat thinking is for looking at logical risks. These probably sound familiar – we're used to the idea of 'pros and cons'. What's important about Yellow Hat and Black Hat, though, is that they are used to separate our assessment. So, rather than saying, 'If I go on holiday, I'll feel really relaxed and happy when I get back, but then again, it's going to be expensive,' I'd first list all the benefits of the holiday, then the risks. Then I'd put the Red Hat on and decide, on balance, what to do. (If you're wondering why the separation matters, imagine mixing equal quantities of yellow and black paint. Looking at benefits and risks together can allow the benefits to be completely overwhelmed.)

Black Hat

- Chemotherapy makes you feel more ill than cancer does

- Chemotherapy may have some pretty nasty side effects

- Chemotherapy will keep me 'out of my life' for longer

- Chemotherapy may not be necessary, if the cancer has completely gone, so I'd be putting myself through it all for nothing

- Chemotherapy drugs are toxic and can themselves cause cancer

Yellow Hat

- Going through chemotherapy will make me feel I've done everything I can to stop cancer from recurring

- Chemotherapy takes place over a relatively short space of time

- Chemotherapy side effects don't last forever

- Because I am young in cancer terms, if cancer does recur it is likely to be aggressive

- Chemotherapy boosts my 10-year survival rate from 69 per cent to 86 per cent.

Red Hat decision

Better safe than sorry.

So, it was agreed: Chemotherapy would start on 31 December 2008. Yes, New Year's Eve. Still, as Lou pointed out, at least I knew I would feel rubbish on New Year's Day, unlike everyone going to a party and imagining that they'd only have two glasses of wine then switch to water. Alan and I went out for dinner on the 30th December, our New Year's Eve Eve celebration. And then it began.

TUESDAY, 30 DECEMBER 2008 [ABRIDGED]: A VISION

Think about the last time you cried. Something happened – maybe you saw something, heard something, walked into something, or even thought about something – and before you knew it, there were tears.

If you stop and think about that for a moment, you'll realize that what makes you cry is not the event (with the possible exception of the walking-into) but of the thoughts it sets off. I usually cry when I see my first snowdrop, and it's because snowdrops remind me of my late Grandma, who loved snowdrops, and despite her chronic rheumatoid arthritis would bend down to 'ring the bell' of the first snowdrop that she saw every year, to bring luck. The event triggers the thought, and the thought triggers the physiological reaction, the tears. The same happens when we smile, or laugh: trigger-thought-physiological reaction.

Athletes understand the power of the mind in affecting behaviour, and use it to their advantage. As far back as 1956, the Russian Olympic team took 11 hypnotherapists with them to the Melbourne Games to help them with visualisation. Linford Christie, after running the fastest 100 metres ever, said, "The Olympics is the pinnacle of every athlete's career. They said I was too old but I did it. I had practised in my mind and saw myself do it". Footage of David Beckham at the age of 9 shows him playing football in a Manchester United strip, telling the camera he is going to be a professional footballer.

What has all this to do with me and cancer? Well, I am using visualisation in preparation for chemotherapy, tomorrow and every three weeks from tomorrow for six cycles. I have visualised what's going to happen. First I did it after getting into a relaxed state, sitting quietly, just before going to bed and when I woke up in the morning, until the visualisation became so strong and clear that it's running all the time in the back of my mind, a bit like 'The Chicken Song' did after I saw a clip about *Spitting Image* on TV over Christmas. Let me tell you about it.

Here's what happens in my vision. Alan and I walk to the hospital, relaxed and calm. We arrive on the chemotherapy unit and go through all of the details of the treatment. I sit in a big comfortable chair and have a cannula put into my arm by a nurse who is so expert that I hardly feel it. (I made a decision early on in this whole process that I was not going to be bothered by needles. There's no point. It would be like a squirrel being bothered by nuts.)

Then the chemotherapy drugs arrive, and I hold the bag in my hands, and as I do so I feel gratitude that this treatment is available to protect me, and a quickening of my heart as I realise that this is where my long, happy future starts. I imagine that the bag is struggling to contain a great ball of warm, pulsating light.

The bag is connected to the cannula and the drugs start to flow into my body. I sit back, close my eyes, and visualise light pulsing through me as these drugs course through my system. I feel light, and calm, and take deep breaths. When I breathe in, I think of health, and when I breathe out, I imagine that anything in my body that isn't good for me is being expelled. I imagine that in my body, when the drugs find a stray cancer cell, it explodes like a firework in the night sky, and is gone forever.

I have been through this visualisation so often now that it has become more of a reality than the horror stories that I was so attached to when I first realised I needed chemotherapy, and that scared me so much. I'm visualising the aftermath too, of few side effects and going about life as usual, and posting on this blog about how well I am.

[...]

I'll let you know how it goes.

WHAT CHEMOTHERAPY IS

Nerve gas, essentially.

During the Second World War, medics found that any cancer that was exposed to nerve gas shrank dramatically. (What people with tumours were doing being exposed to nerve gas is a question outside the scope of this book and, very possibly, any level of compassionate human understanding.) And so chemotherapy was born.

OK, I'm oversimplifying, but essentially, all chemotherapy has developed from this simple finding. And what chemotherapy does is this: it races round the body in search of fast-growing cells. Two things make cancer cells dangerous: the fact that they multiply and grow really, really quickly, and the fact that they aren't programmed to die, the way that healthy cells are. So a tumour can grow rapidly, and in doing so it hijacks the body's resources in order to feed itself. (Essentially, a cancer is like Audrey II from *Little Shop of Horrors*. Without the singing.) When chemotherapy finds fast-growing cells, it destroys them. So, the theory goes, if there are any cancer cells hanging about anywhere – and you can get a million of the little blighters on the head of a pin, so they're not always easy to spot – chemotherapy will get them. It sounds like an elegant solution. Until, that is, you think about what else is fast-growing in the human body. Hair cells are fast-growing. Nail cells are fast-growing. The cells of the digestive tract, from mouth to anus, are fast-growing. The cells that line your nose and your sinuses are fast-growing. The soft tissue inside your teeth is fast-growing. The cells of the bone marrow, where white blood cells are made, are fast-growing. And as yet, chemotherapy can't tell the difference. So it destroys them all.

BAH! THINKING 🐉

Questions for your oncologist about chemotherapy

1. Why do you think chemotherapy is a necessary option for me?

2. What are the implications if I don't go ahead?

3. Which drugs will you prescribe? What does each do? Why these ones?

4. How many rounds of chemotherapy would you suggest? Why that many? Could I consent to half now and see how I get on?

5. How and where will the chemotherapy be delivered?

6. What help is available for side effects?

7. Is there anyone I can talk to who has had the same treatment?

8. What will I have to be careful of during chemotherapy?

HOW CHEMOTHERAPY COMES

There are many different types of chemotherapy drugs, and they are given in different combinations – called 'cocktails' – according to the cancer being treated. Sometimes it is given every three weeks, sometimes every week, sometimes every day, for three months, six months, a year, forever. Sometimes chemotherapy is administered before surgery to shrink a tumour to a size where it can be more easily operated on. Sometimes it is given as a safeguard to try to ensure that a cancer doesn't come back, sometimes as a way of trying to eke out the last few months of a failing life.

I was prescribed a fairly standard treatment: six rounds of a FEC cocktail every three weeks. (More about what FEC is in a minute.) The theory is that three weeks gives your body time to rebuild everything that's been destroyed ... except the cancer, obviously. So my routine was: clinic and bloods on Monday, chemotherapy on Wednesday, unless the blood tests showed that the white cell count was not sufficiently high to risk another round of chemo – which never happened to me. Then home to recover, being sure to be extra careful around days 10–14 after treatment, as this was when the immune system was particularly low and so even the most everyday of infections or bugs could become life-threatening very quickly. And then it all started again.

The drugs go straight into a vein, so treatment begins with the ritual of The Finding Of The Suitable Vein. This perfect vessel must be accessible, large enough to handle quite a broad catheter, and the nurse must be able to draw blood back out through it, which (I think) is a way of checking that the needle is in properly. If the needle isn't in correctly, then chemotherapy can make its way into the surrounding tissue, where it will burn through the flesh. To complicate things further, the longer chemotherapy goes on, the worse state the veins get into, and if you have had lymph nodes removed, then that arm cannot be used at all. The first time I had chemotherapy, it took seven goes and two hours to find a vein. This was due entirely to my poor-quality veins, and not poor-quality nursing: In fact, one of the nurses trying to get the needle in sat in front of me shaking her head saying, 'I am so ashamed,' and she was more upset than I was.

This all took place on a day unit, full of comfortable chairs for patients. (They were supposed to recline but I never got one that did anything when I pressed the buttons.) There were not-so-comfortable chairs for relations. There was lots of natural light. There was a not-quite-tuned-in radio playing. There were always more people than there were chairs, and more pouches of chemotherapy than there were drip stands, and more drugs requiring a pump than there were pumps, all of which lent a kind of make-do-and-mend, spirit-of-the-Blitz, street-party atmosphere to proceedings. But I always struggled with the public aspect of chemotherapy. Although being able to talk to other people and see what is going on does have benefits, there is something I found odd and unsettling about sitting in a room full of strangers while a nurse poked about in my arm or cross-checked my drugs. I suppose I felt that my treatment was an intimate and personal thing, so I didn't really want strangers to be watching, any more than I would invite people to come in from the bus stop outside to watch me shave my legs. Once I sat next to a man having a blood transfusion, and I really felt that that was something I shouldn't be seeing, somehow. Another time, an older lady having chemo for the first time burst into tears, and I wished for her that she could have done so in an environment in which she was more comfortable.

The F in FEC stands for 5-Fluorouracil, which goes in through a syringe, and made my heart flutter. E is Epirubicin, which is also administered by syringe, and is red, and makes all body excretions for a few days afterwards a peculiar shade of orange. I didn't especially mind this. What I did mind – in fact one of my Top 5 Freak-Out Things through all of my dance with cancer, although I didn't say anything at the time, just sort of curled up and cried inside – was being told to use condoms because the chemotherapy could make my excretions so unpleasant that they could cause discomfort for Alan. I mean, eugh! I'm pulling a face just thinking about it.

The Epirubicin goes in first, because it is, basically, the most nasty, so needs to be injected while the whole vein-catheter thing is at its strongest. The C is Cyclophosphamide, which goes in via a drip, and made the inside of my nose and my sinuses ache immediately. I could feel the pain trace a figure-of-eight round my forehead and face. Then the vein is flushed with saline. The whole thing takes a couple of hours, although some chemotherapy cocktails can take anything up to seven hours to be administered.

And then it goes to work.

CHEMOTHERAPY THINKING

If you look up 'bloody minded' in a dictionary there's a good chance you'll find a picture of me there, right between my dad and my brother. People lining up to tell me how awful chemotherapy was going to be made me (a) determined it wouldn't be and (b) really cross. (Try this. Ask everyone you know, for a whole day, to say to you, 'You're going to have a terrible headache when you get home.' Go home. See what happens. My guess is it will involve ibuprofen.) Oh and (c) determined to prepare properly.

I started to use visualizations. Every time I thought about chemotherapy I thought about it as bright, golden light, flowing through my body, meeting any lingering cancer cells and exploding them into a little sparkle of dissipating brightness. And I thought about it all the time. Deliberately I thought about chemotherapy morning, noon and night, and I thought about it healing me, and I thought of it as a force for good.

Every time I went for chemotherapy, I took the tray with the drugs in it and I closed my eyes, and I held my hands over them and I tried to make a connection, to think of the drugs as something I was welcoming into my body.

The big mental step I felt that I took was making the decision to stay in the world. I didn't stop working, for a start. Although I didn't work all the time – maybe only three or four days in every three-week cycle – and even though I got a hell of a lot of stick from my Macmillan nurse about it, still being able to do what I did, and what I loved, reminded me that I wasn't really losing my grip on my life. It wasn't easy. I took taxis distances I wouldn't normally think twice about walking. I delivered a lot of training sitting down. I ate crackers and biscuits and drank milk constantly to keep on top of the sickness. I had to find a way to explain to people I'd just met that I was being treated for cancer, but despite all appearances to the contrary (hat indoors, robot arm) I was fine, and I had to do it without making people feel sorry for me.

And I tried to bring my usual approach to life and work – my enquiring mind, my desire to understand, my need to look beyond what is presented to me – to my treatment. This did not make me a favourite of some of the people who treated me, but it helped me to stay in control.

MY DRAGON ARRIVES

One day I went for a massage, and I talked to the therapist about how I was using visualizations to ease my symptoms and support my treatment. I told her how they had been useful to start with but didn't seem to be helping much any more. She said, 'Visualizations need to change. Perhaps think of an animal coming to protect you.' Later that day, I idly watched my son playing a game which featured two knight-types having a sword fight while riding dragons. And suddenly, there she was: my own dragon. She seemed to ping forth out of the very air, fully formed and full of all the feistiness and strength I couldn't manage.

She stayed with me through all the difficult times. When I was having chemotherapy, she became huge, and she sat behind me and wrapped her wings in front of me, a curtain carapace, so I was in my own protected space. During those long afternoons when I was at home by myself and the phone was quiet she'd fly figures-of-eight around my head, telling me I wasn't alone. When I was sleepless, she would sit on my bedpost, awake too, and I didn't feel quite so low. When I went shopping, and was struggling to know what to eat, she'd perch on something that I would then buy and enjoy. When I was calm and happy, she'd be wheeling in the sky overhead, distant but ready. When I blogged about her, she'd sit nearby and preen.

What I loved about the dragon was that, although my mind had created her, she wasn't an effort in the way that other visualizations were. I thought of her more as something that my subconscious brain had made to help me out. Since my dragon appeared, I've spoken to people who have had big blue butterflies, or bears, or cats, or wise old men accompany them through their dances with cancer, all doing much the same as my dragon did for me.

BAH! THINKING 🐉

Preparing for chemotherapy

Chemotherapy can be physically and mentally traumatic, and the more you can do in advance to get yourself ready for it, the better. This list is some of the things I did – and some of the things I wish I'd done.

1. Decide what you want to do about side effects. Everyone you see explains them to you, over and over again. They do it for the best of reasons – to inform you, to prepare you, because if they don't explain them properly you might sue them – but it's tedious and depressing and makes you expect that things will be horrible. If I'd thought of it, I might have asked not to be told about side effects, and taken the approach that if I had problems I would let the hospital know. I'm not sure that would have worked, though, as it would hardly count as informed consent. So maybe I would have listened to it once, taken all of the leaflets, and then very politely refused to discuss it further. Or maybe I would have asked someone to brief Alan on side effects so he would know what was going on.

2. Think about what you might find difficult, and do what you can to prepare. A big barrier for me was the fact that, according to everyone and their dog, nausea and chemotherapy go together like rhubarb and custard. My problem was the fact that I hate being sick. OK, nobody likes it, but in the scheme of non-life-threatening illnesses I'd take a week of flu, a broken ankle or a urinary tract infection – or possibly all three – before I'd choose to throw up, even once. So having everyone chuck in 'Oh, and of

course you'll be nauseous most of the time' casually at the end of a big list of what they considered to be much worse side effects, threw me into a panic. I had decided on my own that I wouldn't mind needles, and that had worked. But I couldn't manage to not mind the nausea. So I had some hypnotherapy before chemotherapy began, and it worked like a dream. (Well, like a trance, I suppose.) I was cured of my horror of being sick. Just like that. Really.

3. Stockpile good reading, DVDs, jigsaws/knitting/crossword books and phone numbers, so that you always have something to read, something to watch, something to do and someone to call.

4. Be careful who you talk to. Listening to lurid tales about how your colleague's auntie vomited out her own stomach lining is neither necessary nor helpful. You don't have to talk to everyone who wants to talk to you.

5. Get your diary up to date with likely treatment dates, points where your immune system will be low, so you will need to keep away from public transport and crowded areas, days when you will be strongest and could go and do something you enjoy. It seems amazing, when I look back, that for the duration of diagnosis, surgery and chemotherapy, I never caught so much as a sniffle, though this was due in part to the good offices of my friends, who were kind enough to steer clear (and to tell me that they were doing so) if they were even slightly unwell while I was having chemotherapy.

6. Sort out some comfortable clothes to be your chemotherapy wardrobe. You might be sitting around a lot. You might gain, or lose, weight. Be kind to yourself in what you wear. That doesn't mean you should consign

yourself to a grey marl tracksuit with gravy stains down the front. (Unless you want to, of course.)

7. Visit the chemotherapy unit before your first treatment. I did this, and even though I showed up unannounced, the Matron of the unit dropped everything and showed me around. He explained the procedures and showed me where treatment would happen. It was a room filled with ordinary-to-grey-looking people with drips coming out of their arms. A radio was playing, there were big windows, and there was a level of chatter and to-ing and fro-ing that I found reassuring: no deathly hushes, no tears.

BAH! THINKING

Finding your visualization

Get comfortable and quiet. Close your eyes. Breathe, and think about breathing. Breathe more slowly, right down into your body, until all you are thinking about is your breath and how it fills you.

Think about chemotherapy drugs, and think about them in your veins, helping and restoring you. Imagine how they are going to make sure you are healthy and well for years to come. Wait, and see how your mind sees chemotherapy. Maybe the drugs seem like little cancer-seeking missiles, whizzing through your system looking for cancer cells and destroying them. Maybe they are friendly Pac-men, munching up anything that shouldn't be there. They could be dazzling shards of healing light, or tiny pantomime horses trampling on the nasty, or ninja warriors or smiling faces, or erasers rubbing out what shouldn't be there. It doesn't matter what they are, so long as you can imagine them doing their work.

Sit quietly for a while visualizing the drugs going to work. When you are ready, open your eyes.

Once you know what the chemotherapy looks like to you, practise seeing it go about its work every day.

If the image of chemotherapy stops working, do the visualization again. What works to begin with might feel less useful later.

THURSDAY, 1 JANUARY 2009 [ABRIDGED]: CHEMOTHERAPY – DANCE 1

I tried to take good care of myself from the moment I woke up on my first day of chemotherapy. Alan and I had celebrated New Year a day early, so went to bed late, slept late, and had breakfast in bed. I took a long bath (not that I ever need much encouragement to do that) and put on a cheerful top (butterfly print), a necklace we bought in Turkey in May that makes me feel warm and glad every time I wear it, and the earrings Alan gave me for Christmas. (I put on all the other clothes that would normally go with, in case you're wondering. Not the weather for partial nudity.)

[…]

(I went to the bathroom before we started the chemotherapy, and allowed myself a little moment of feeling really, really scared. Then I looked myself in the eye in the mirror, and said, "Brave. Strong. Supported." Which I was. As well as a little bit really, really scared.)

[…]

Two and a bit hours, two soaks in a sharps bucket [to help the veins pop out], and seven attempts later, we were ready to go. Manjula found the vein in the end, and when she realised that she had done it, watching her face was like seeing the sun come up.

I'd visualised holding the chemotherapy in my hands, but as there were three big syringes and a bag to go in, Manjula held them in a tray so I could put my hands over them. I thought this might feel a bit silly, but I experienced a profound sense of gratitude to these drugs that are giving me life. I saw them as light, and I thanked them, and we were off.

I closed my eyes, sat back, and felt the light and healing flow into my body. I started to inhale 'well' and exhale 'ill' and then the oddest thing happened. A sort of slide show began in my head. I saw myself in Finland with my family this time next year, cosy and warm in a snowy heaven. I saw Alan and I in a place that I knew was Barcelona, where we've always wanted to visit. I saw myself back at work, and felt all the satisfaction that work gives me, and I saw myself here, at my desk, satisfied in a different way. I saw myself watching the Northern Lights, and swimming in a jewel-blue sea (not at the same time). I saw myself walking on a beach and felt the salty, fresh air in my body. I saw myself with my children, my godchildren (except we're godless), my friends, holding a baby who'll be with us next month (not mine). And I was drenched in a feeling of well-being. It was as though my mind was reminding me that this is just a blip in the long, happy life that I am already embarked upon. This will sound really odd, but I may well remember sitting in that chair as one of the happiest moments I've experienced.

Anyway. We walked home via M&S food, and called people to let them know I was OK, and drank tea and ate crumpets. By now it was 7pm and I was shattered, so napped for an hour, got up, went back to bed... and started to feel sick and headachy. The headache was the worst thing, probably because I wasn't expecting it. The nausea wasn't a patch on morning sickness, so I propped myself up on some pillows and ignored it. 3am and a meditation on my iPod (a meditation I'd downloaded to my iPod, not a big think about my iPod) and I was off to sleep – 8.30am, awake, and feeling absolutely fine. Really. Breakfast, anti-sickness meds, blogging, I'm off for another bath.

One down, 5 to go.

SIDE EFFECTS

I'm going to talk about side effects for a bit now. These were mine. They don't have to be yours. Please skip forward if you want to.

Side effect 1: Hair loss

This wasn't anywhere near the issue for me that I thought it would be. First, I look damned fabulous in a hat, if I do say so myself. Secondly, hair loss is such a given in our cultural concept of cancer that I think I was getting used to the idea from the second I was diagnosed. And I must admit I was a little bit curious to see what I would look like bald. So I embraced the idea of hair loss as much as I could. Before

Christmas, I had my hair cut really short – or what I thought of as really short. Before the second round of chemotherapy, when the hairs at the front of my head started to loosen, Alan took me to the barber for a Grade 4 head shave. When my hair started to go, I took regular photographs and posted them on my blog, which I saw as a kind of public service, I suppose. I knitted a lot of pretty hats. I rejoiced in not shaving my legs and armpits.

I'm not suggesting for a moment that losing hair is a fun activity that everyone should try on a rainy day. Now and then I had an attack of feeling unfeminine, but Alan soon chased those away for me. My scalp itched and I woke cold in the night. I felt odd wearing a hat indoors. And I became obsessed with other people's hair. I learned how to spot a wig from 40 paces (as long as I had my contact lenses in). I longed to stroke the hair of people sitting in front of me on the bus. I became incensed whenever I saw someone with scragged-back-into-an-elastic-band unappreciated hair, and I found it really difficult to follow film plots or news items because I was so easily distracted by the hair of newsreaders, characters or, in one case, a corpse. And waiting for it to grow back seemed to take forever. But hair loss was not that much of a big deal for me.

WEDNESDAY, 28 JANUARY 2009: MINDING AND NOT MINDING

I find it strange that I don't really mind the dance with cancer itself that much. I haven't done a lot of 'why me' or 'not fair' (although others have on my behalf, and it breaks my heart to see it) – maybe because my life of late has been so immersed in love and happiness that, perhaps, it's time for a little rain to fall. Maybe because, cancer and all, my life is still immersed in love and happiness. Maybe it's because, assuming that some sort of illness will befall me at some point, an operable breast cancer at a time when the medical community can knock it on the head pretty effectively, and when I am otherwise well, fit, young, financially secure, and with a support network as solid as a rock, is not a bad way to do it.

There are things that I do mind. I mind the tiredness, the breathlessness (I walked up three flights of stairs on Tuesday, and had to stop because I was literally – and this is a correct use of the word literally – keeling over), the 'out of body' feeling in the few days post-chemotherapy; it's as though I am my own puppeteer, steering myself jerkily through everyday life. I mind the amount of time that's being sucked into sitting in waiting rooms and walking hospital corridors, and the fact that when I tell someone I'm OK they look at me a bit sideways. And I mind the PICC line. I'm trying to think of it as my bionic arm, my unaccustomed plumbing, my highway to a bruise-free life... but I mind it. I really do. And with it I mind not being able to have a proper bath or go swimming. (Not being able to play golf, squash or tennis is just fine.)

More than anything, I mind the fact that my family and friends are anxious and worried and saddened by my dance with this disease, and I wish I could make them realise how much I don't mind it; how it's just a little thing that's teaching me a lot and giving me a lot, however much I wouldn't have chosen it, and however much it bugs me sometimes. It's heartbreaking to see your parents and your children upset; but as we continue through this dance I think we are all starting to mind a bit less.

Side effect 2: Stripped-out gut

The stripping of bacteria from my gut, from top to bottom, was a pain in the backside, and everywhere else. My mouth was sore, and for a while I didn't go anywhere without a flask of hot salty water to rinse it with at every opportunity. I had truly awful heartburn, and the tablets I was given to combat this made me feel sick and bloated and headachy. I couldn't eat any of the foods I loved and craved – soft fruits, rich stews, anything with cheese – and so my digestive system became confused and I became even more constipated than the lack of bacteria was already making me. (Chocolate, fortunately, was OK after the first few days of the chemotherapy cycle, but is not noted for its laxative qualities.) Eventually, I stopped trying to work out what I wanted to eat and tried to eat a little of everything that was put in front of me, and that worked better, but for someone who loves to cook and bake and spend time around the table with near and dear, this one was no fun. No fun at all.

BAH! THINKING 🦎
Food and chemotherapy

This is not one of those what-to-eat-to-bring-perfect-nutritional-balance-and-healing sections. There are others who do that way better, and way more convincingly, than Stephanie 'pass the custard' Butland is likely to. This is a list of things that I ate when my digestive system was in meltdown. As someone who normally eats a lot of fruit, the fact that I struggled to do so threw me completely. Not only did I become constipated (a most under-rated ailment), but I felt slightly out of kilter. Here is a list of the things that I mostly ate, and which might not upset your system too much. You'll be able to add your own, of course.

1. Pasta with olive oil. This is simple, it's not obviously bad for you (unless you put the oil on with a ladle), and it's unlikely to upset your stomach. And if you struggle to eat fruit and your bowels lock as a result, the bulk of the pasta and the oil can help to get things going again.

2. Rice pudding. Easy to swallow and coats the digestive tract, so if you have heartburn (another much under-rated complaint) it may relieve you. I found that custard and chocolate milk did much the same thing. Mind you, I put on half a stone during chemotherapy. And I can't look at a bottle of chocolate milk without feeling queasy now.

3. Ginger tea or peppermint tea, which settle the stomach, are easy to prepare (especially if you're a bag-in herbal tea drinker like me) and smell lovely.

4. Nuts and dried fruit, which are nutrient-heavy and not acidic, so I found them easy to digest. The acid in most fruit made them a no-no for me. 'Bananas!' I hear you cry, and I'm sure you're right, but I'm not a fan. In fact I can't see why anyone would put something that smells like that in their mouth ... but if you can, do.

5. Pea soup. Easily digested and, frankly, a bright change from all the pale stuff I was eating. Other soups, too.

6. Dopiaza. I know that, given the list so far, a spicy dish seems to fly in the face of all that I'm saying, but at around day seven of the cycle, every time, I'd have a huge urge for dopiaza from the Indian takeaway across the road. I'm not sure why, although I think it could be that the dish is made with a lot of onions, which are traditionally an antiseptic, so perhaps my body was craving what it needed.

7. Cornish wafers. These are buttery savoury crackers, and I was on about a packet a day at one stage. 'Eat little and often' is the great sickness-avoiding mantra, and these were the little things I ate often. Ned used to come home from school via the supermarket and pick up a couple of packets every day.

8. Gingerbread. Need I explain?

THURSDAY, 12 FEBRUARY 2009 [ABRIDGED]: CHEMOTHERAPY THE THIRD

To the hospital yesterday afternoon, with Scarlet's blessing ringing in my ears: enjoy today, and be filled with light. Alan and I had had a quiet, relaxed morning, and I had knitted, breathed and thought myself into a calm state. (I wasn't exactly not calm, but there were a few little demons around, reminding me that just because the first two rounds of chemotherapy had gone OK it didn't mean the third one would.) We walked to St George's through a clear, crisp afternoon.

It all went very smoothly – the drugs were there and ready, so no waiting, and [...] they were administered quickly and easily, by the lovely Rachael (who was relieved to see that I didn't have my camera this time). There were two tiny side effects – the second of the drugs made my heart go all a-flutter for a few minutes (not entirely unpleasant) and the third one makes my sinuses ache for about 20 minutes. It's the oddest sensation – I can actually feel it trace a loop around my forehead, nose and behind my eyes as it makes its way. (The first drug also has a side effect – it makes my wee go pink – but I wasn't sure you'd want to know that.)

And leaving the hospital, I saw my first snowdrop. It wasn't the prettiest of snowdrops, and it's hardly surprising, growing as it was in a flowerbed between the inner ring road of the hospital and the entrance, so being in a prime place for both pollution and being trodden by people taking a shortcut. No, it was bowed, and ragged, and a little bit grey. (Quite appropriate for me just now, then.) But it was a snowdrop all the same, so I rang its bell for luck, and I felt the way I always do at this first sign that spring will come, and life begin, again. In fact I felt it all the more.

A snowdrop is also my direct link back to my Grandma, who died in 1992 after dancing with rheumatoid arthritis with grace and humour and the minimum of fuss for many, many years. When I come to think of it, 'enjoy today and be filled with light' could have been her motto – although what she did was closer to filling others with light, always fully involved with her family and keen to support, and love, and knit for us all.

So when I left the hospital I was buoyed up and happy, with Alan beside me, my Grandma around me, spring in front of me and all of your thoughts behind me.

No wonder that what I feel more than anything right now is blessed.

Side effect 3: Insomnia

It really doesn't take more than two or three nights of fewer than eight hours of unbroken sleep to turn me into a borderline psychopath that even I am afraid of. Steroids, given to counteract feelings of nausea brought on by chemotherapy, make it difficult to sleep. The need to go to the loo often, as the body processes out all of the drugs and deals with the after-effects, means broken nights. The inevitable anxiety can't help with a good night's sleep, and the reduced physical exercise that tends to come with treatment (or at least came with mine) means that the muscles of the body aren't tired in the usual way, even though the nasty-drug-processing organs may be working overtime.

So I was tired, but in an odd sort of way, I guess because my body was so busy dealing with the onslaught of chemotherapy that it didn't have much time for doing the usual stuff. Perfectly understandable, really, but I've never been too tired to think before, or felt as though I was watching my thoughts slowly make their way to the surface of my consciousness, like the beads of lava (or whatever it is) in a lava lamp.

Tiredness is one of those symptoms which, if mentioned to an oncologist – or my oncologist, at least – gets a response along the lines of, 'Oh dear, oh well', and a subtext of, 'Please don't bother me with trivial and peripheral issues when I am terribly busy trying to save your life.' Eventually I solved the problem by going to see my GP, who gave me sleeping tablets to take on the few nights after chemotherapy. It really was that simple. I don't especially like sleeping-tablet sleep – it's a little like being switched off and switched on again, and I have no awareness of the fact that I've been asleep like I do on a normal morning – but it's a thousand times more preferable than some of the long, sad and frightened nights I had without them. Not to mention the snappy sleep-deprived days, mostly spent hoping for and dreading night-time. And trying the patience of my family.

Side effect 4: Breathlessness

Being breathless is quite scary. Getting breathless walking from your sofa to your kettle to make tea is downright depressing. Because being breathless can be a sign of deterioration of the heart muscle, it's taken quite seriously as a side effect. Once it had been found that there was nothing wrong with my heart, it was dismissed with those decidedly un-magic words, 'It's a side effect. It will get better once chemo stops.' Not helpful words, and all the more annoying when you find them to be true.

THURSDAY, 5 MARCH 2009 [ABRIDGED]: CHEMOTHERAPY 4: WHAT GOES DOWN, MUST COME UP

[...] As I walked to the hospital I was fighting tears, especially when I crossed the railway bridge and had to stop every five steps or so in a hope that the pain involved in climbing steps would ease. (It didn't.)

As soon as I met Alan at the hospital, the tears came. I wasn't really scared or upset so much as worn right out, and I couldn't help myself. We had some lunch and meandered up to the chemotherapy unit. I took a deep breath and decided to be brave and strong. This lasted right til Amy, one of the chemotherapy nurses, came over and said 'How are you doing, sweetheart?' Then there were more tears. Not sobbing, just a constant flow. And not the kind of tears that cry themselves out; the tears that multiply the more attention that you give them, and the kinder people are to you. So I was in big trouble.

We had to wait an hour to see a doctor, and I'd said that I didn't want to have the chemotherapy until I had. I guess I was holding myself hostage: I knew the medics wanted me to have the chemotherapy more than I did so I had a better chance of not getting the brush off if I hadn't had the chemotherapy. (Yes, I know there's a hole in that argument that you could drive a circus train through.) That hour passed in a bit of a daze; I slept, and wept, and I think I did both together for a bit because I opened my eyes at one point and realised that the tears had run down my face and neck, been channelled through my cleavage and come to rest in my belly button. Nice. Oh, and at one point someone came along and did reflexology on my feet. Highly recommended (but perhaps in a different context).

Lovely Dr Laura [...] came to talk to me and she was great. She listened to what we had to say then had a chat with Debbie, the oncologist I've seen most often (and not on Monday). They agreed that the pain is an unusual but legitimate side effect of chemotherapy and prescribed anti-inflammatories and something to protect my stomach lining from anti-inflammatories, as a first step; if they don't work we'll go on to something else. I took the first dose, and then we went on to the chemotherapy.

I like to hold the chemotherapy before it's administered, and see it as something that is welcome in my body, and will heal me. Yesterday, although that was my intention, what came into my head was a sort of plea along the lines of 'please help me. I can't cope with much more of this.'

By this point, my internal reservoir had dried up, and Alan, Amy and I chatted as the chemotherapy went to work. Side effects were minimal; the second drug, which sometimes makes my heart race, didn't, although the third one, which causes an instant ache in the sinuses, did. (Amy says that in Australia, where she is from, chemotherapy patients suck on an ice lolly when having that drug to minimise the effect. We'll take one in next time, and it can sit in the freezer with the cold caps until we need it.)

I walked out of the chemotherapy unit feeling like a different woman. [...] Walking home through the frosty air, I couldn't believe how much better I was. A sleeping tablet meant 8 hours of sleep with only one break, so that's an improvement too; on the last three rounds of chemotherapy, I've struggled for 4 uncomfortable hours of sleep a night in the few days afterwards.

This morning continues well. I'm up and blogging and the aches and pains, if not gone, are not debilitating.

Side effect 5: Nausea

I felt sick. I felt sick most of the time. Feeling sick became like background noise, like your deaf neighbour's too-loud TV that you stop noticing after a while.

Side effect 6: Aches and pains

This was my Bonus Symptom. This started sometime after the third cycle of chemotherapy, and it got steadily worse. To begin with, it was an intermittent, fluey, generalized ache that made it uncomfortable to either be still or move around, but over time it worsened, until it reached crisis point after the fifth round of chemotherapy. I felt the kind of pain you'd get from being laid under a concrete slab with a rugby team sitting on top of it. (Not that this has ever happened to me, you understand; I'm speculating.) I ached, and I cried, and we had a hell of a job getting help from the alleged out-of-hours service at the hospital, but we eventually got some slightly more serious painkillers than paracetamol. (The next time we saw the oncologist, she said she wouldn't have prescribed them because they 'are not necessary for FEC patients'. You may begin to see why she isn't on my Christmas card list.) I'm aware that I've reframed a lot of my experience and tried hard to take the good from what did happen – it's part of my strategy. But those few days were beyond awful. I went to bed every night thinking that tomorrow would be better, and it wasn't. I woke up to find I was already crying. I watched my husband, always calm and capable in a crisis, helpless and upset in the face of what was happening to me. (This was what's known in our family history now as the Terrible Weekend.)

HOW TO HELP: What to do when someone you know is having chemotherapy

1. Don't make assumptions. Chemotherapy does not equal perpetual illness, just like cancer does not equal death. If you're not sure whether your chemotherapy-undergoing friend can/would want to do something, just ask them.

2. Go with them to appointments. Keep them company. Even if they insist that they are quite capable of talking to the oncologist/having a blood test/having chemo on their own, don't let them. I know whereof I speak, because I sometimes did the oncologist/blood test bit on my own, and when I did it always brought me down. I'm not sure why I did it. Maybe I didn't want to be a bother. Which is, frankly, one of the most ridiculous sentences I've ever typed, but for people like me who are not used to asking for help, someone taking time off work to sit in a succession of waiting rooms with you seems like a lot to ask. Save us from ourselves and insist.

3. Take them some food. You don't have to turn into a super-chef and rock up with a gourmet home-made feast. Go to the supermarket and buy some good bread and soup, or something that goes into the oven and comes out ready to be eaten straight from the tray with a spoon.

4. Lend them some DVDs. A box set of something with no more than 30-minute episodes was ideal for me, because on days when all I felt like was lying round watching TV, I had the attention span of a gnat, so I couldn't concentrate for very long.

5. Bring magazines. I don't usually read magazines, but chemotherapy robbed me of my interest in a lot of books. I think it was because what I was mainly doing was caring for myself, and novels require you to care about someone else, at least for the four hours or so that you are reading them. So, for the first time in memory, I didn't feel like picking up a book. I did, however, quite enjoy a couple of hundred words about why dinner parties are the new trips to the cinema, or being introduced to the baby of a celebrity I'd never heard of via very few words and lots and lots of shiny pictures taken in unfeasibly tidy houses. (I also managed the odd edition of *Private Eye*, so I didn't turn into a complete intellectual amoeba.)

6. Work out their schedule. Put the days when their immune system is lowest – and therefore they are less likely to be out and about – in your diary, and arrange to visit. (Cancel if you have a cold.) The weekend before the cycle starts again is a good time to suggest seeing a film or going out for lunch.

7. Call in the middle of the afternoon. Philip Larkin wrote about 'the hollows of afternoons', and during chemotherapy I discovered exactly what he meant. On a bad day, 3 p.m. can feel like the time where the whole world is busy doing something, and whatever it is doing is so absorbing that it has completely forgotten you. People often said to me, 'I was going to call but I thought you might be sleeping.' I'd rather have been woken by a phone call than got through the afternoon without it: even though you know you are thinking of me, when you decide not to call just in case you disturb me, I'm none the wiser.

8. Ask questions and make comments. (Nice comments.) You might think that pretending that wearing a hat indoors is completely normal behaviour will spare the feelings of the newly bald. It won't. It may seem that pretending that chemotherapy isn't happening is the right thing to do. It isn't. (Or at least, it wasn't for me.)

9. But also be prepared to talk about other things – including yourself. Chemotherapy can reduce the world to something small and dark, as we move from consultation to test to treatment and round again. Feeling like part of the wider world is a good, good thing. The importance of being able to help and support someone I love didn't go away just because I was having chemotherapy, and I'd have been devastated if anyone I knew felt they couldn't talk to me about their own difficulties because I was having chemotherapy.

10. I had so many conversations with people that went like this:

Them: How are you?

Me: Fine, thanks.

Them: How's the chemo going?

Me: Nowhere near as bad as I thought, actually. I tend to have a couple of down days, but I'm mostly fine.

Them: That's good. [Here comes the part you must never, ever say.] Of course, the side effects get worse as they go on, don't they?

Now tell me, what is the point of that last remark? Up until then it had gone so well. And yes, it might get worse. But if it does, you've not helped by pointing it out. And if it doesn't, you've worried someone who has, frankly, quite enough to worry about right now.

BAH! THINKING

Positive action

A list of Green Hat ideas about what to do if chemotherapy gets you down is a good thing to prepare in advance. Here's some of my thinking.

1. Think of, or do, something that pleases you. Or talk to someone who does.

2. Hang out at a knitting shop. (Or any shop that pleases you, where you will meet like-minded people who can take your mind off it all for a while. I'd aim for a shop with chairs or sofas. Bookshops also work very well.)

3. Meet friends during their lunch hours.

4. See films on your own in the afternoon. Honestly, it's liberating. You get to choose everything: the film, the seat, the sweets.

5. Recognize, and ask others to recognize, when you are feeling sorry for yourself, and make a determined effort to stop.

6. Play whatever you think of as fantastic music very, very loud.
   And conversely ...

7.   Let yourself be down if you need to be, for a little while. I was absolutely determined not to feel sorry for myself, and I was absolutely determined not to be an invalid. Looking back, I'm not sure this was the right thing to do. I think the odd day of staying in bed rather than making myself be out there in the world, all eyes and teeth and 'See how well I am!', might have been as useful. I think admitting that I didn't feel up to much might have done me the world of good.

Before I was diagnosed, my friend became pregnant, and asked me to be her birth partner. Two cycles into chemotherapy, I did just that. Not only that, I did it overnight between two days of working, with a couple of hours of sleep on a mattress on the hospital floor in between. So, bang in the middle of what was supposed to be the worst period of my life, I made a memory that is up there in the top 10 best things I've done ever.

Peripherally Inserted Central Catheter: Crossing the line

THE LINE

A Peripherally Inserted Central Catheter (PICC to its friends) is a line that runs from a vein, usually in the arm, up to just above the heart. It allows drugs to be delivered into the body safely and without fuss via a port on the outside of the vein, which remains in situ for as long as the PICC is needed. One of the chemotherapy nurses suggested that I get one after the first seven-attempts-to-get-a-line-in round of chemotherapy. The nurses were concerned that (a) it wasn't much fun for me – or them, I suspect and (b) because veins tend to deteriorate during chemotherapy, if it wasn't easy to get a line in the first time, the chances of being able to do it in the future were slim to zero. So a PICC seemed to me to be a sensible idea. Although I'd decided not to mind needles, being cannulated isn't really my idea of a high old time, but I went to have it fitted.

I thought it would be straightforward. Well, that's not true: I didn't think about it at all. I didn't research the procedure, so I rocked up all set for something little more than an ultrasound-aided cannulation, with (I think I imagined) some sort of dinky tap/valve thing, possibly designed by Terence Conran, on the outside of my arm. I didn't get what I expected. When the person doing the insertion got out a startling array of needles and wires and put thick wadded blankets under my arm, I started to realize what I was in for. The procedure wasn't painful once the local anaesthetic was in, but there was a lot of shoving and a great deal of blood. (As soon as the line goes in, the vein is, in effect, open, but then the port has to be fitted to it, and until it is, the blood just keeps coming. I don't really mind blood, but I prefer it in smaller quantities. I swear there was enough to make a black pudding.) And I wasn't too keen on having the port, in effect, sewn onto my arm. (This was referred to as 'being held in place by a couple of stitches', which may be a more medical way of putting it, but comes down to the same thing.) And there was much more medical hardware on the outside than I'd fondly imagined there would be. I walked home crying and shaking afterwards – I'd thought it would be a quick bit of nothing, and had gone on my own – and I waited to get over it.

TUESDAY, 20 JANUARY 2009 [EXCERPT]: A WHOLE LOT OF HOSPITAL

This little lot [the PICC line] means no swimming, bathing only with one's arm out of the water, and showering when wrapped in clingfilm (not all of me, that would render showering pointless – just the arm). It means having dressings changed every week and wearing an elastic tubular bandage all the time. But what I am finding most difficult, and what had me crying after the procedure, on the way home from the hospital, when I got home, and now as I write this, is the idea and the feeling that I am now a kind of invalid. I see my scars as part of my physical landscape now, and a badge of survival and sign of life. Hair loss is more interesting than traumatic, and an opportunity for many pretty hats. But this little lot I am struggling to reframe in a positive way, maybe because it's more than I bargained for, maybe because it's not part of my body however altered, maybe because it feels so cumbersome and looks so darned ugly.

I know this is insane, and vain. Alan says that this is the mark of being well, not being ill, and of course he is right. I am trying to focus on the positives: at 7 attempts per intravenous treatment for chemotherapy and herceptin, I've saved myself 154 digs into my arm and 44 hours, as well as 22 lots of blood tests. And I now need to go shopping for pretty long sleeved things… So it's not all bad. Not all bad at all.

And that's before we get to the bigger pluses, like the fact that there are such things as chemotherapy and herceptin and PICC lines at all, and that cancer is not going to dance me to death, as it might well have done a couple of generations ago.

I know that I need to keep focused on these positives…. it's just that right now they keep slipping away from me whenever I move my arm with its unaccustomed new cargo.

FRIDAY, 6 FEBRUARY 2009 [ABRIDGED]: A GATEWAY TO HEALING

We [Gosia (the hypnotherapist) and I] got on to the PICC line. We spent a lot of time talking about why I didn't like it – I can be quite eloquent on that theme – and we nailed it down to four main areas: it's ugly, it stops me from doing things, it's alien, and it's a constant reminder of treatment for cancer.

So ... we discussed the best way to treat me. One option was to hypnotise me into loving it, but we agreed that that wasn't really the right thing to do – it felt a bit inauthentic, and I had a momentary vision of me explaining all about it to people on the bus, cutting the arms out of all my long sleeved things so that I could always see it, giving it a name, refusing to have it removed ... Then we talked about hypnotising me into not minding the fact that I mind about it, but that didn't feel quite right either. Then I remembered something that Alan said on the day I had the PICC line fitted, when I came home in tears saying that it made me into an invalid, and he said I could try to see it as something that is making me better. (Which I did try to do, but as you know if you've been reading, that didn't go terribly well ...) So Gosia and I focused on that. We decided that the PICC line is a gateway to healing.

I can't tell you very much about the hypnotherapy itself as I was so relaxed that I don't remember much of it ... but I can tell you that as I type I'm wondering what on earth I was so bothered about. I've barely looked at, or thought about, the PICC line since the session, and when I have, I haven't thought about it directly, rather

I've had a mental image so strong that I've been able to draw it – well, not so much draw it as copy it down.

[...] And with the mental image comes a feeling of peace, of calm, of wellness. I feel the way that I'd feel if I'd just been for a lovely walk in the country on a sunny summer day, and I'd come to that gate, and I knew that there was a cafe serving cream teas on the other side of it.

(Just to clarify: I don't look at my arm and see a wooden gate surrounded by flowers in it instead of the PICC line – that would be scary. I just have the thought of my little picket gateway to healing, and all of the positive feelings associated with it, in my mind. Which is much better.)

So ... I think I'm over the PICC line. Thank you for your patience. Let's move on.

So, I learned to live with it, but that didn't mean I didn't love having it removed. And I wasn't thrilled when, later, during herceptin treatment, I had to have it back because my veins were even less accessible than they had been at the start of chemotherapy. But I'd learned, and I did better.

TUESDAY, 12 JANUARY 2010 [ABRIDGED]: READY AS I'LL EVER BE

Of everything I've been through in my dance with cancer, the PICC challenged me most, and upset me most, and was the most difficult to come to terms with. (Yes, worse than hair loss.) So deciding to have it back, after the last herceptin debacle, was a difficult step to take. Needs must, and all that, but imagine choosing to go through something that really hurt you all over again, and you'll know it hasn't been an easy call to make.

But, having made the decision, I knew I had to make a better job of preparing myself than I did last time. So that's what I've been doing. (Obviously, I know what I'm in for this time, so that helps.)

First, I did some research, to see whether a Hickman line (into the chest) would be better than a PICC. I decide that it wouldn't be… so I felt as though I'd made a choice, and the PICC was a better option. (As well as being a better option than being repeatedly stabbed with a needle every three weeks, of course.)

Then, I didn't request the appointment until I was ready to. I knew it had to happen, but I waited until I'd got my head round the whole idea, as much as I thought I was going to. This meant last Friday, when I emailed Rachael and asked her to organise the appointment for the morning and herceptin for the afternoon.

Then, I asked Gerri to come with me. Not only does Gerri knit and make me laugh, but she's also genuinely interested in the medical side of things, which helps me to be engaged by the process and distracted from the implications.

Then, I contacted Gosia, the hypnotherapist and transformational coach I first met via The Haven, and booked a session with her.

Then, I had lots of big bubbly baths. (And I also treasured every moment I had [had] in the water in Egypt.)

Yesterday, I had a session with Gosia. What I love about working with her is that she doesn't just go, 'OK, you're worried about having a PICC line, let's hypnotise you and make you believe that the PICC line is your best friend and you won it as a prize and everyone is jealous of you'. Gosia finds out what's behind the fear, the difficulty, the worry, and she works to help with that.

Last time I had a PICC, part of my distress was all to do with feeling like an invalid when I was striving so hard to believe and make myself well. Gosia helped me to see the PICC as a gateway to healing, and it was a huge help.

This time, the PICC felt like a step backwards. It felt like a sign that my dance with cancer will go on and on and on forever. It felt like an intruder into my body, and I have always been uncomfortable with the fact that it sits so close to my heart. Gosia and I explored this, and we decided that the PICC, rather than being something that got in the way, was something that was going to make my treatment easy and effortless and over sooner. We also talked about it as an outward manifestation of how life could be easy too. She put me under (or whatever the hypnotherapy term is) and we replaced the fear and worry with a sense of welcome and ease.

Now, I'm aware that might sound a bit bonkers to you, and of course you are welcome to feel that way. But I have to tell you that shortly afterwards I had an email from someone expressing their sorrow and sympathy that the PICC line was back.... and I was genuinely bemused, along the lines of 'why would anyone be sorry about a PICC line?'. I think it's powerful stuff. Of course, it may be powerful simply because I believe it's powerful, but frankly, so long as it works, I don't much care.

As a result of my session with Gosia, I feel calm. I feel ready. I feel something that I can only describe as being a deep sense of home.

[…] I've also prepared by finding and buying a PICC protector, so I will be able to have showers and baths in relative ease. (According to the site I'll be able to swim, too, but I might see how the baths go before I fling myself into the pool.)

Tomorrow, I will wear clothes that I love (I think the shiny red shoes might be coming out again), take some really nice knitting with me, and remember how lucky I am. Between now and then, I will be running over the process in my mind, again and again and again, and as I do I will be imagining it going really smoothly, really easily, really well.

And, never one to miss a shopping opportunity, I'll probably buy myself a little present too. […]

I think I'm ready. Have I missed anything?

de Bono's Checklist of Current Thinking

This is a Lateral Thinking™ tool that I wish I'd thought to use during the PICC times: it would have been, I think, the difference between trying to lace up your basque in the dark, or doing it with the light on.

Like many of de Bono's tools, this one is beautifully simple. It asks you to examine what you think about something by considering your dominating ideas, your assumptions, the boundaries, essential factors, and avoidance factors.

If I'd done this with the PICC, this is what I might have found.

PICC: Checklist of current thinking

- Dominating ideas: PICCs are for invalids.

- Assumptions: A PICC goes into the arm. The procedure is uncomfortable. PICCs are ugly, unwieldy and make life difficult. Except for when it comes to getting drugs in or blood out.

- Boundaries: PICCs are for the period of intravenous treatment and/or problematic veins. PICCs need to be kept clean and accessible. PICCs can't deal with large volumes of liquid at high pressure (e.g. when having a CAT scan). PICCs require short or loose sleeves.

- Essential factors: A PICC should work. It should reduce pain, difficulty and time in hospital.

- Avoidance factors: The PICC shouldn't cause, pain, infection or major inconvenience.

I think that if I'd done this little bit of thinking before I'd gone into hypnotherapy, we'd have got where we needed to much quicker.

BAH! THINKING

What's behind the problem?

What the PICC taught me, more than anything else in my dance with cancer did, was that sometimes, what seems to be the problem is not the problem. Here's a way to see what's getting in the way for you. You don't have to do it all in one go: sometimes leaving it and then coming back to it is a more effective way.

Find a quiet place, a blank sheet of A4 paper, and a pen.

Take the paper and put it long side down (landscape) in front of you.

On the extreme right-hand side of the paper, write a few words that describe the difficulty you are having.

Ask yourself, 'Why does this bother me so much?' or, 'What's the problem with this problem?'

Write down what comes into your mind, to the left of the original difficulty.

Then ask, 'Why is this important?'

Write down the reason to the left.

And so on, until you feel as though you've got to the heart of the problem.

Now, if you read from the left of the paper to the right, you have a whole chain of thinking that leads to the apparent difficulty.

Then ask yourself how you can get help with the cause that you've identified as the real reason for the difficulty. It might be something that simply vanishes because you've identified it; it might be that a conversation with a friend helps you to get it out of your system; it might be that help from a counsellor, therapist or hypnotherapist is what you need.

Take action.

❦ ❦ ❦

Enough, already: Calling a halt

THURSDAY, 26 MARCH 2009 [ABRIDGED]: CHEMOTHERAPY 5: SUNSHINE AND SHOWERS

I don't know how the weather was where you were yesterday, but it was gloriously unpredictable in this little corner of London. During the course of the day, I got rained on, hailed on, blustered about.... and the sun shone so brightly that I cracked open my sunglasses for the first time this year!

Internally, my weather was similar.... I was really aware of how my poor state of mind and body going into my fourth chemotherapy meant that the side effects felt tough and it took longer to pull myself around. So this time I was determined to treat myself well, and prepare myself positively, for the fifth round.

[...] on Tuesday I took it easy and tried to focus on:

the good things in my life

the fact that I can be treated and will be well again (and I'm not sorting my clothes into bin bags so that nobody else has to do it)

only two more chemotherapy treatments to go.

I cooked a lovely meal for us on Tuesday evening, and was feeling very positive… until I had a little pre-bedtime wobble and a few tears. Alan reminded me how well I'm doing (more tears) and I had a big whine about how hard it all is. We decided that the best course of action was to pack me off to bed, and by 9.30 I was spark out and dreaming.

We had a new strategy for chemotherapy day. Last time, Alan went to work and I stayed at home on my own, working myself up into a state of misery all morning (the aching was at its worst) before we met at the hospital, when it was really difficult for Alan (or anyone else) to sort me out. This time, Alan had a day off and a meeting in Kingston in the morning, so I went to Kingston with him, and headed for a book shop and the yarn department in John Lewis for an hour. We met up again after his meeting, had a coffee, then went back to John Lewis (I wasn't quite done with the yarn… so many possibilities!), then headed for home. Lunch was crusty bread and soft cheese, and it was feeling as though the morning had done its job of keeping me occupied and getting ready with a cushion of nice things for the aftermath (knitting, books, tasty things from Waitrose).

But after lunch, as Alan prompted me about leaving for the hospital, it all went a bit miserable again. I had a real 'I don't want to go' moment, complete with tears, and if that resonates with your experience of trying to get a small child to go to school, that's funny, because it pretty much resonates with my own experience of being a small child and not wanting to go somewhere. (Usually I did want to go to school though. That's me all over. Wasn't too keen on caravanning holidays.)

Anyway, Alan pulled me together, and off we went. There was a bit of a wait for the chemotherapy drugs to be ready. (They have to be freshly made up shortly before they are given. I like to think that this is because they could rot through anything they're put into, given the chance.) Then Sophie came to collect us.

Sophie is a fully qualified nurse who has just been through her training to specialize in chemotherapy/oncology. She was an absolute delight. She did everything perfectly, and with consideration and friendliness. She didn't even bat an eyelid when I asked to hold the drugs before they went into me.

My visualisation for the drugs changes every time, and this time they felt like energised, bouncing bubbles beneath my hands; I saw them coursing round my body and popping where they were needed, exploding anything that was thinking about becoming cancerous (although I am pretty sure I don't have any of those anyway). As I closed my eyes, I could see my dragon perched on the side of the tray, looking very beadily at the drugs; I think there was a bit of a 'good cop bad cop' thing going on, with her having a serious word about how we could do without the side effects.)

After that it all went smoothly. The first drug never gives me any problems going in. It wasn't until we were walking home that I realized that the second one hadn't either – usually it makes my heart beat faster, and I tend to fall into a doze. The third one usually makes my sinuses ache, but we took Amy's advice (she did the chemotherapy last time) and took in an ice lolly to try to alleviate this particular side effect.

It worked – in that I wasn't aware of the acute ache marching in a figure of eight around my face – although the dull pain afterwards is still there.

The aftermath is OK so far. When we came home, I thought I wanted to go to bed, although it turned out that I didn't after I'd got there, so I got up, knitted for a bit, and Alan and I had supper, most of which I couldn't manage. I did manage to stay awake through The Apprentice (who wouldn't – it's like watching a multiple pile up in slow motion, over and over – you just can't tear your eyes away) and then headed off to bed properly, plus sleeping tablet.

My night wasn't brilliant – quite a lot of 'drifting just below the surface of sleep but not completely rested' thing – but I've had worse. And today I'm tired and achy and my face hurts – but it's been worse.

As I write the rain is rattling on the Velux window above me. My guess is it won't be long until the sun comes out.

FRIDAY, 27 MARCH 2009: YESTERDAY'S GONE

... and I'm glad to see the back of it. What a day! Definitely my worst post-chemotherapy day so far.

Firstly, I didn't sleep well, despite the sleeping tablet, so I was tired when morning came around. I had a bath and dozed on and off through the morning. A bath and a doze usually perk me up no end, but not yesterday. Along with the usual methods of support and sympathy were a couple of people – trying to be helpful I'm sure – pointing out that hasn't time flown since I started chemotherapy on New Year's Eve? To which the answer is – NOT HERE IT HASN'T.

I had a nice big cry, followed by a little sleep, and then Ned and Joy came home, which was lovely. An attempted walk to Tesco with Alan had to be aborted early, making my jog round the park on Tuesday seem like an impossible achievement. I rang my mum in tears but she managed to cheer me up.

The rest of the day was characterised by little cries and attempts to nurture myself, including doing a bit of knitting, which is always a good thing, and reminding myself that (a) this is a day that I never have to have again and (b) I'm nearly there and (c) I am going to get better, unlike some people dancing with cancer.

Sleep was better last night, so I am going into today from a better position than I was in this time yesterday. And I keep reminding myself that the chemotherapy side effects last only a few days, so by Sunday at the latest I will be a mostly functioning adult again. That's the plan, anyway. Watch this space!

SUNDAY, 29 MARCH 2009 [ABRIDGED]: BLOW BY BLOW

My blog post on Friday morning was, as it turned out, pretty optimistic. The sun didn't shine. I cried and cried. The pain got worse, but we couldn't really work out whether it was physical pain or all of the emotional stuff that inevitably goes with this dance, finally being released now that we are almost at the end.

Alan rang the hospital and spoke to the lovely Barry, matron of the day unit, who put us on to Caroline, the counsellor, who was also lovely. Joy dropped in on her way home from school: she'd had a rough day too, so we snuggled up on the sofa and comforted each other […]

As Friday wore on, it became clear that the physical pain was increasing. I took sleeping tablets and painkillers, went to bed, and slept a little better, thinking 'surely the worst is over now'. But Saturday morning greeted me with the feeling of being crushed under a slab of concrete (with cancer dancing on the top). The painkillers didn't work. The steroids didn't work. The warm bath didn't work. The big cry didn't work. The dragon tried to help, but there was only so much she could do. Alan held my hand.

At 11.30 am we rang the hospital. I dozed on and off, I think. At 1.30pm, we rang the hospital again, and Alan spoke to a nurse on the oncology ward, who took all of my details, and said that the oncologist on duty would get back to me within an hour.

She did, and she was lovely, although when I heard the words 'there isn't a magic pill' I would have cried if I'd had any crying left. Still, we agreed that my pain was at an unacceptable level and that she would write up a prescription for co-codamol (which is morphine based so given out with caution), get it from the pharmacy, and it would be ready to collect by 6.30pm. Not ideal.... but very obviously the best that they could do, so I settled in with my knitting and [TV] ... I found that as long as I didn't move too much the pain was tolerable. I was also trying to bear in mind that the pain I was going through was a walk in the park compared to others'.... and that five days tends to be the maximum for post chemotherapy effects, so I was more than half way through this one, and almost at the end of the whole thing.

[...]

Alan rang the ward as agreed at 6.30pm, to be told that the prescription was not ready and may not be ready til the morning. He put on what I recognised as his 'enough is enough' voice and very calmly pointed out that this was unacceptable and disappointing. He was then told to ring back at 9pm; he agreed, and said that if the prescription wasn't ready, then we would need to come in to hospital via A&E to try to get help that way. Despite my self-administered pep talks, I was in despair at the thought of another day like the one I'd just been through.

[...]

Anyway, at 9pm Alan rang back to find that the prescription would be ready in 20 minutes, so he went to get it, and I went to bed, and when he came back I took the painkiller and the sleeping tablet and when I woke up around 5am everything was starting to feel much better. The slab was being winched off, slowly but surely, and another dose of co-codamol had me up and showered and dressed. I'm both relieved – pain is sooooo underestimated! – and infuriated that something that could have helped sooner was only given to me after 3 days, despite my earlier aches and my meeting with the oncologist on Monday.

Anyway. Here is the plan.

1. Make complaint to hospital about lack of support from out-patient services (but not staff on duty) and lack of information to patients about what they can expect if unwell outside office hours

2. Take Alan to next meeting with oncologist as supporter and anti-fobbing-off device

3. Make sure I have 5 days' supply of steroids and co-codamol in my hand before consenting to further chemotherapy

4. Get re-focused on the positives: I am alive and well and chemotherapy is nearly over

5. Go out for lunch (I'm doing that first).

CALLING A HALT

After the Terrible Weekend, my thoughts turned to the next round of chemotherapy. The side effects had got steadily worse, to the point of excruciating pain and breathlessness. (At one point I even Googled 'glamorous walking stick', which tells you a lot about me. Yes, I'll have a walking stick if I have to, but only if it's gorgeous and matches my outfit, thank you very much.) I started to wonder whether I would ever recover from chemotherapy. I started to believe that another round might actually kill me. And I started to think about whether doing it again was really such a good idea.

I can imagine that, if cancer has a grip on your body and is waiting to take you over, that any level of pain in the name of a cure, or even a little more time, is acceptable. But from the moment I had the results from my surgery, I have chosen to believe that I am cancer free. So for me, chemotherapy was an insurance, a way of protecting my future – but a protection that I never truly believed that I needed. (Maybe you will read that and see it as wishful thinking or burying my head in the sand. Maybe you're right.) And I went along with it, until it came to the point, after the Terrible Weekend, when it seemed to me that the Actual Chemotherapy was much more of a danger than the Hypothetical Cancer.

I talked to Alan, who, having watched me go through such a wretched time, was happy for us to think about not having the final chemotherapy. Ned and Joy, too, were supportive. The harder sell was going to be to the rest of my family, who I suspected would make the equation 'not completing chemotherapy = much more likely death'. Ned, Joy and I were going to visit, so I told them a little about how I was feeling before we set off.

SUNDAY, 5 APRIL 2009 [ABRIDGED]: WHAT WOULD YOU DO?

Since the last round of chemotherapy 11 days ago I've had a growing feeling of unease about the treatment. Understandable enough, you may think – nobody's going to feel great about subjecting themselves to something so uniquely and relentlessly nasty – but I've come to realise that there's more to it than that.

What it comes down to is this: I really feel that the potential side effects (and their long term implications) of another round of chemotherapy are going to outweigh the potential benefits. The breathlessness and sinus pain are things that the doctors can't seem to tell me whether will get better or not. They seem to have established that there's 'nothing wrong' with my lungs and heart which just makes me all the more anxious. I can foresee a situation where I limp through the rest of my life unable to walk up stairs … which is all well and good if the alternative is to be dead from a recurrence of breast cancer. (Despite everything, I haven't quite forgotten to be grateful that I can be treated.)

Given that the tumour was removed in its entirety, the lymph nodes were clear, and chemotherapy is essentially part of an insurance policy, I'm wondering whether 5 rounds of chemotherapy + radiotherapy + herceptin rather than 6 rounds of chemotherapy + radiotherapy + herceptin is going to make a great deal of difference. (As far as I am concerned, I have been cancer-free since the lumpectomy on 18 November.)

I'm also trying to listen to my body's own wisdom and instinct. I have been waking every morning with a very clear thought: 'Don't. Do. This. Again. It's. Not. Right. You'll. Regret. It.' Again, hardly surprising given the way the last 11 days have been, but there's an imperative to it that's hard to explain: the nearest I can come to describing it is the urge to push when you are giving birth (not a lot of use to those readers who haven't, I'm afraid). The fact that my body has done so well so far only makes me take this all the more seriously.

Let me be clear: if this was just about immediate side effects I'd be quite happy to put on my grown-up girl's shoes, take a deep breath and a lot of drugs, and get on with it – but my instinct is, very strongly, that another round of chemo will do more harm than good, both short and long term.

Sadly, no crystal ball is available. I could sail through the final round of chemotherapy. I could decide not to go ahead and be cancer-free forever, or develop another breast cancer in 5 years. I could have the 6th round and be cancer-free forever, or develop another breast cancer in 5 years. Whatever I do, I'll never really know whether it's the right thing.

DE BONO'S CONSEQUENCE AND SEQUEL

Here's another tool that would have been really helpful if I'd thought to use it. (I am infuriated by books in which the protagonist does all the right things all the way through. It's bad in fiction, worse in non-fiction. There's no danger of that happening here.) Consequence and Sequel simply asks you to set some relevant timescales – three months, one year, 10 years – and think about what your view of the decision/problem/thinking at hand might be at each of those points in time. So, if I am thinking of buying a car I can't really afford on my credit card, then I might feel fantastic about it in three months, as I drive around in my shiny new toy with heated seats and a retractable roof. (Hell, I might even heat and retract at the same time, I'm feeling so recklessly ecstatic.) In a year, the novelty of both the car and the payments might have worn off, and I might be starting to regret my decision. In 10 years, there's a good chance I'll still be paying for the car, as well as paying ever-heftier bills to keep it on the road.

A lot of the trouble and distress at this stage of my dance with cancer came from everyone having a different perspective in time. I was firmly rooted in the here and now, feeling ever more tired, more breathless, more in pain. Many of the people who love me had an eye on my future, so their view was much more long term. Consequence and Sequel would have given us an easy way to understand this. We did it the hard way.

We arrived in Northumberland to a lot of well-meaning chats about taking the long-term view and just getting through this one because you have to think of the future. My brother gave a convincing hypothesis of what was happening in my body to make me ache and be unable to breathe, and why it would quickly pass once the last round of chemotherapy was over. I think lactic acid was involved. (After this, Ned said to me, 'You know, Mum, whatever you decide to do about chemotherapy, I'll support you.' It was a little bit of shelter in a storm of well-meaning, well-motivated, loving pressure. The dragon stayed very close by, too.)

On the Sunday evening, I 'fell over' – not literally, but this had become our expression for what happened to me when my body had had too much. I was pale, I was shaking, I could barely breathe or stand. Joy put me to bed. My parents were shaken: they were seeing first-hand what they had only heard about by phone before.

The next night, I went to bed early, but was woken by toothache shortly after midnight. After a couple of hours of fruitless attempts to get back to sleep, I got up, went downstairs, and cried. I cried loud and I cried long. I cried wishing for someone to wake but no one did. After a good hour of solid sobbing – and I wasn't just crying because of the toothache, or the aching, but for my changed life, my forced confrontation of mortality and fear, my worried children, my bald head – I called Alan. He was as gracious and sweet as a husband woken by a distraught and virtually inconsolable wife at 2:30 a.m. could be: he virtually consoled me, in fact, and I got a couple of hours' sleep before facing another day and getting my tooth treated.

Now, having a toothache when you are having chemotherapy is not as simple as going to the dentist. Oh no. Especially not if you get it around day 12 of the cycle. Pain = likelihood that chemo drugs are attacking inside of tooth. Tender mouth = injections to be avoided. Although that's largely irrelevant because low white cell count = reduced immunity making even tooth extraction risky in infection terms. That's before you add the frisson caused by the danger that, once bleeding starts, it can't be stopped due to lack of clotting factors in the blood. The upshot of all this was that my dad and I spent the day at the dental hospital waiting for the dentists in Newcastle to talk to the oncologists in London, and came away with some whacking antibiotics and crossed fingers. Fortunately, the antibiotics (or the fingers, or both) got to work and the tooth pain was on the way out within 24 hours.

Something had changed, though. When the question of the final round of chemotherapy came up again, there was no more 'Be brave, be strong, just one more and it will all be over.' The mood in the camp became 'OK, we can see this is destroying you.' We talked about what to do. My surgeon had always asked me to contact him at any time with any question. I sent him a long email, asking his view on the dangers of cancer coming back after five rounds of chemo versus the dangers of giving chemo to someone who was disintegrating. Within 15 minutes I had a one-line answer: 'I can see you in clinic tomorrow.' My dad put me on a train in Newcastle, and Alan got me off it at the other end.

The meeting was the most surprising I have ever been to. We went in hoping for information that might help us to make what seemed like a really scary decision. We came out with the decision practically made for us; White Hat can do that sometimes. We were told that each round of chemotherapy destroys 90 per cent of any cancer cells present, so the first two rounds really do most of the work. We were told that for women who had had the results from surgery that I had, 95 per cent would have no cancer remaining in their body so chemotherapy was irrelevant, though necessary, because for the other 5 per cent, it would probably save their lives. We were told that, although I would recover from the side effects of chemotherapy, it was fine to stop having it – not having the sixth wouldn't make a great deal of difference.

We drove back to Northumberland in a daze. It was over. It was over. It was over.

And it was time to start on the next bit.

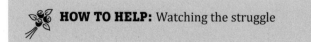 **HOW TO HELP:** Watching the struggle

I often thought, even during the grimmest parts of my dance with cancer, that it must be worse to watch someone suffer. Here are some ways you might help, if your loved one is in difficulty.

1. Don't assume anything. Ask a lot of questions – gently, but keep going until you feel you really understand.

2. Once you think you've understood, ask about what you can do to help. Could you gather more information? Speak to a doctor on their behalf?

3. Try to look after the mundane. If your loved one is having a terrible time, not eating and not sleeping will only make the terrible time more challenging. Heat soup. Make tea. Run baths. It really helps.

4. If your loved one is making a decision that you don't agree with, be very careful about how you challenge them. Remember that their perspective is different to yours.

5. Be the cool head. Ask: Is this a decision you have to make now? Is this truly urgent, or is the emotion/exhaustion making it feel urgent?

6. Remember that your role, above all, is to support. There may come a time when you have to watch someone do the thing that you wouldn't do if you were them. Remember that you don't really know what you would do in their situation. (I'm pretty sure that, if I were Snow White, I would have seen straight through the crone with the impossibly shiny apple.) Be gracious.

Cancer and relationships: It's not just you

I don't think that a dance with cancer changes you *per se*. I think it tests you, and in the process of being tested, you might change. The same is true of relationships. Relationships change not because you have a dance with cancer but because the process of a cancer diagnosis and treatment tests those relationships. Sometimes it tests them to destruction. But – in my experience – not often.

MONDAY, 16 FEBRUARY 2009: HOW THE WORLD SHRINKS

I realised something this weekend, following on from my last post: I realised how carefully I've been cared for, how beautifully looked after, since this dance with cancer began. Of course I always knew that I wasn't doing it on my own, and I've been grateful for every bit of help, from cups of tea in the morning to flowers to the fantastic and supportive comments on and via this blog, to drug treatments that my grandmother's generation could have only dreamed of.

But yesterday I watched my fairy goddaughter Evie pushing her truck of bricks around, and I got some perspective on what's really going on here. Evie is nearly one and she really thinks she can walk, but here's what happens. First, someone sets up the truck for her and makes sure there's a clear run. Then they stand her behind it. Then she pushes the truck until it hits a wall, and she sits down, maybe a bit more suddenly than she was anticipating. But before she can get too worried, someone picks her up, turns her round, and sets her off again. And she goes, without a look back, and with 'I can walk! Look at me walking!' all over her face.

That's pretty much me. 'Look at me! Coping with breast cancer! Handling treatment!' And I kind of am, in that I'm putting one foot in front of the other. But in so many other ways I'm not [...] that's how it has to be sometimes: you have to give over control and accept the process. And I'm grateful, so grateful, to everyone who is keeping me going here; turning that truck of bricks around and setting me off again, and giving me a round of applause every time I make another lap.

It's hard not to feel that I ought to be doing better/ more; I felt a bit overwhelmed just walking to Tesco on my own on Friday, and that's not me at all. Except, on Friday, it was. And that's OK. My world is a small one right now, and I'm learning to live with that, because a small world is what I need at the moment. A safe home, fantastic family, loving friends, supportive colleagues, excellent treatments, and plenty of knitting. Everything else can wait.

Many things affect your relationships while you are dancing with cancer. You may have preconceived ideas about how people should behave around you. Your family and friends will almost certainly know someone else who has danced with cancer, and that experience – including whether that person lived to tell the tale or not – will inevitably colour the way they behave towards you. The chances are that your treatment for cancer will go on for a long time, and during that time life will wend on for your friends: babies will be born, people will die, marriages will begin and end. (Hopefully, your treatment will not go on for so long for that to be the same marriage.) Some people will be better at supporting some parts of your dance than others.

THE BELOVED

I don't think there's a word for the way Alan has been during my dance with cancer. (And I mean that in a good way.) He has supported me brilliantly, never treated me like a patient or an invalid, listened and done things differently when I needed him to. But more than that – he has done all this without making me feel any less myself, or any less of a woman. He has waited while I took a rest after walking up four stairs, stayed within reaching distance while I bathed and showered, warmed rice pudding up for me at odd times of the day and night, without ever letting me feel that this was anything other than perfectly normal marital behaviour. (Which of course, in one light, it is.)

There were times when our sex life suffered, but that was more to do with me being in bed and asleep by 9 p.m. for weeks at a time, and being prone to agonizing and unpredictable cramp, than it was to do with anything more fundamental. One night after sex, not long after surgery, I asked Alan if he felt differently about me now. I suppose I was hoping for, 'Of course not, darling, you'll always be beautiful to me,' or similar. What I got was, 'Do we really have to have this conversation?' which did much more for me than the other answer, from page 22 of 'How to reassure your wife that she is still attractive after something unpleasant has happened to her womanly bits'. (It also made me realize that I wasn't being truthful in asking the question. I knew he didn't feel differently. I think I'd been reading too many leaflets.)

 HOW TO HELP: Some tips for navigating your relationship through cancer

1. Don't assume that you know how your partner feels/what they want/what they need. Ask them. You are both still the people you were pre-diagnosis; you are both still adults.

2. Sit down and have a conversation about how to approach the dance with cancer. I wanted Alan to keep working but reserved the right to ask him to take time off/work at home when I needed him to. Your partner might need you within arm's length at all times, or feel that Carrying On As Normal will support him or her more.

3. Find a way to tell each other when you need help. Alan and I had an expression ready prepared: throughout our relationship when one of us has been struggling with something and needed the other to look after us, we've asked, 'Can you carry the torch for a while?'

4. Look after yourself and look after each other. Rest. Eat good food. You are both going through a strange and difficult time. Be kind.

5. Find someone you can talk to about what's happening for you. Yes, you should be able to talk to your beloved, but being able to talk to someone else too is important for you.

6. Be prepared to overrule your loved one when need be. There have been times when Alan has persuaded me to eat or sleep even though I was sure that wasn't the right thing to do. It was. Assert when you need to.

7. Keep doing the things that you do as a couple. If you usually go to the cinema on a Thursday, then do it. There's no reason to put everything in life on hold.

8. Have times when you decide and agree not to talk about cancer. Whether it's a mealtime or a weekend, give yourselves a break.

9. Keep telling each other that you love each other.

THE CHILDREN

When I think about my dance with cancer, the most pain and the most pride comes from thinking about my own children, who have shown themselves to be mature, compassionate and generally all-round magnificent. (I know everyone thinks that about their children. But in the case of mine, it's true.) I have had to let go of my urge to protect and to pretend everything is all right, all the time. It took me a long time to work out that the correct answer to the question, 'How are you doing, Mum?' was, 'I feel terrible, actually,' rather than, 'Fine, darling, just a bit tired.' The first, Ned and Joy could do something about – a cup of tea, a hug, a chat – whereas the second left them feeling, I think, unsatisfied and a bit cross, because they could see straight through my whole 'Me? Fine. Fine! Never better!' schtick.

SUNDAY, 14 MARCH 2010 [EXCERPT]: ON MOTHERING SUNDAY

I know it's mandatory – indeed, it's a biological imperative – for mothers to think that their offspring are fabulous. But I'm sure regular readers know enough to agree that Ned and Joy really are. My children have been part of my dance with cancer with depths of maturity, understanding, patience, compassion and humour that have amazed me, and I thought they were pretty amazing to begin with. They've shown me that I can trust them with the big stuff and I've learned that if I can overcome my natural instinct to protect them from unpleasantness they will support me and we will all be better, closer, stronger for it. I would have given anything for them not to have had to experience cancer with me, but I can't imagine how I'd have done it without them. Thank you, Ned. Thank you, Joy. You're the stars in my sky. And you choose a good present, too.

There are some other children in my life, of the teenier variety. At the time of diagnosis my nieces were eight and five, my godson was three and my goddaughter a babe in arms. I found being around them all a real gift.

Partly, I think, because although they could all (except baby Evie) understand about me being unwell, they didn't have the great weight of experience and cultural education that tells us that cancer is a Terrible Thing To Be Feared Above All Else. They just knew I was poorly. So they treated me just the same as they always did.

WEDNESDAY, 29 JULY 2009 [EXCERPT]: PERKED UP

Louise, Ellis's mum and my best friend these 20 years, has always treated Ellis like the intelligent soul he is, so he has known about the cancer for as long as we have. (Please be reassured: not in graphic detail. Along the lines of Auntie Stevie having something in her that shouldn't be there, and she needs to have an operation and special medicine to make it go away.) And he has reacted with love and heart-lifting honesty. When I had my PICC line he was very distressed by it. I explained what it was for, and showed him where the special medicine would go, and said it was a kind of robot arm. Ellis's reaction? 'If I was a robot, Auntie Stevie, I would NOT have THAT in MY arm.' Fair dos. Similarly, when my hair was just starting to come back, and everyone was being very encouraging about how good it looked, Ellis said, 'I just think you look a bit scary.' Which was exactly what I thought every time I looked in the mirror.

HOW TO HELP: Some tips for cancer and children

1. Agree with the parents how you are going to approach cancer with the children you are close to. Use the same language as the parents: whether it's 'cancer' and 'chemotherapy' or 'not very well' and 'special medicine', be consistent.

2. Don't try to hide things. Children can tell. That's not to say you should take your five-year-old niece through the minutiae of radiotherapy side effects, or give an eight-year-old child nightmares by explaining precisely how terrible you are feeling right this minute. But be essentially truthful.

3. Decide what you can do to maintain your relationships with children. You might not be up for five hours at the adventure playground throughout treatment, but maybe you could go out for ice cream.

4. No matter how bad you feel, remember birthdays and other special days.

5. Keep talking to the children in your life about what's happening for them. Your dance with cancer is only a very small part of their landscape.

6. Make sure that you give children the opportunity to talk to you about what's going on, if they want to.

7. Don't make them.

8. If you are talking to adults when children are around, don't assume the children aren't listening, or don't understand. In fact, assume they are listening and do understand. Just to be on the safe side.

FAMILY

Chemotherapy waiting rooms are usually pretty much of a muchness. Quiet. Weary. Grey. People recognize each other and exchange a few words as they wait. Now and again it's different, usually because there is someone who is especially nervous or afraid, so they talk more and start desperate conversations and, although I always wanted to reach out and take their hand, and hold it hard, and say, 'All will be well,' I never quite did, because – well, because you don't, do you, although you should.

One day there was a woman just like that in a waiting room. She was talking, fast and hard, to and at anyone who caught her eye. She wasn't unpleasant, but she was obviously in a rotten state – and you have to be in a pretty bad way for it to be noticeable on a chemo ward. This woman – she was probably in her forties – was wearing a wig. It was a pretty good wig, but it was obviously a wig because no patient in a chemotherapy waiting room has a full head of hair, let alone one that's swingy and shiny. Someone commented on what a good wig it was, and she said, in a painfully brittle voice, 'I had to get one because I'm going to stay with my parents next weekend and they don't know about the cancer.'

Now I know, of course I do, that not everyone gets on with their parents. I know that some parents are old and frail. I know that some people feel that they are better off not maintaining a relationship with their family, and it may well be that they are right. But I cannot imagine getting through my dance with cancer without the support of my family, especially my parents, and my Auntie Susan. My parents have listened to me, supported Alan, Ned and Joy, come to stay, come to the hospital with me, and done a thousand small things to let me know that they are with me. Susan has sent me presents and cards, made me laugh, and told me she was proud of me. My dance with cancer reminded me how much family matters.

FRIENDS

Most of my friends were kind and caring through my dance with cancer. But they did it in different ways. Some were really interested in the medical side, while others got a bit squeamish as soon as I mentioned so much as a syringe. Some wanted to Take Me Places and Do Things while others thought a coffee, some nice biscuits and curling up on the sofa was absolutely the right way to go. Some talked directly about cancer while others did everything they could to support me without reference to the c-word.

Part of what I needed to do was to understand which friend did what best. Then I could match the friend to the mood/activity and we would both be happy.

Of course, some friends found cancer too much for them, and drifted free of me. Although it's tempting to be disappointed, I try not to be. It's not as simple as 'finding out who your friends are'. Really what you find out is how comfortable your friends are with cancer. And if the answer is 'so uncomfortable that they can't bear to be around it', then that's sad, but understandable, I think.

MONDAY, 4 MAY 2009 [ABRIDGED]: FRIENDS INDEED

I had a real treat yesterday. Jude had decided that we weren't just going to be glad that chemotherapy was over with – we were going to celebrate that fact. So she organized a 'no more chemo' lunch. How fabulous is that? [The guests were Evie, Jude, Scarlet and Rebecca.] …

These four ladies have been a bedrock of support and love for me over the last six months. Variously and together, they have lunched me, dined me, brought dinner over; listened to me talking about cancer, and allowed me to very definitely not; sent me cards and brought me presents; admired my not-hair, helped me deal with my PICC line, made me laugh, and listened to me whinge, moan and cry; and crucially, introduced me to the novels of Georgette Heyer. (If you're convalescing, there's nothing like the tale of a regency dandy and a sparky heroine, or a pirate with buckles fully swashed pursuing a sultry Spanish maiden, to make the hours fly by.)

Most importantly, to a woman, they have treated me like myself. (Evie has been especially good at that.) No kid gloves, no 'let's not worry her'… I was going to write 'no special treatment' but that's not quite the case. They have managed to treat me in a very special, very nurturing way without ever making me feel an iota less myself; and they've allowed me to be a friend to them too, which matters a great deal when there's so much that you can't do. They have been a place where I am just me, just a part of our network of celebrations and difficulties, good days and bad, giving and taking.

So, it was a huge pleasure to spend a few hours, a few bottles of wine, and some splendid food, with these great friends. We toasted 'no more chemo', and then we got on with the important business of talking about the rest of our lives [...] Which is just as it should be. Thanks, ladies.

DE BONO'S OPV (OTHER PEOPLE'S VIEWS)

There's one thing that causes almost all of the problems I see in my professional life. Yes, really, one thing, whether the people I'm dealing with are CEOs or first-jobbers, whether I'm at a pharmaceutical company or a factory or a government department.

Here's the one thing: It's really easy to believe that everything that we can see is everything that there is to be seen.

Truly. It's almost always as simple as that. When I tell you that we are behind schedule or not good enough or missing out, I am telling the absolute truth, and so if you disagree with me I won't be happy. In fact, I'll try to change your inferior view. Because I have forgotten that the absolute truth is, in fact, not absolute. It's just my truth.

Hence the OPV. de Bono asks us, simply, to consider who else might be involved in whatever we are thinking about before we do it. So, a week on a beach the moment you finish chemotherapy might look like a really good idea from your point of view. An OPV will suggest that you look at that week from the point of view of your medical team, your friends, the travel company ... and when you've done that, your thinking about that week may well change.

BAH! THINKING 🐉
Maintaining relationships

Like so much of a dance with cancer, relationships go better if you take some time to think about what will work best. An OPV helps. Here's some of what I did.

1.   Ask the right person to help you with the right thing. There's no point in asking someone who lives on takeaways to come round and cook you dinner (unless you fancy a takeaway). Lots of people volunteered to come to hospital appointments with me, but one or two who did were really, really uncomfortable when they got there. They'd offered through kindness and the desire to support me, and I was grateful, but it just made for stress for both of us.

2.   Spread the load. Try not to rely on one person for too much of anything. It puts both of you under pressure.

3.   Be clear about what you need. Keep a list somewhere of things you have to/would like to/need to do. Then when someone calls and asks what they can do, you have options to hand.

4.   If you are the one dancing with cancer, remember that life is going on for everyone else. Ask others how they are. Offer what help you can to people in crisis. Even if you can't do what you would normally do for someone having a difficult time, you can still find a way to show them that you care.

5. Realize that some people need to do things, and let them. This goes both ways. I am someone who needs to Do Things, and I'm sure there were times when my near and dear would have loved to have stopped me, but didn't because they understood my sense of frustration at being ill.

6. Agree, or suggest, 'terms of engagement' for the duration of your dance with cancer. You might tell people that you will inform them if there is something wrong, but if not, they can assume you are OK. You might decide that a phone call once a week, or getting together for tea once a fortnight, is the best way to progress.

MONDAY, 8 MARCH 2010 [EXCERPT]: AN ADMISSION

Cancer is like a brightly-lit, high-definition mirror. It shows you every little thing there is to know about yourself, good and bad. It shows you what you do well, what your strengths are, the good bits you didn't know you had. It reflects the areas of your life that work, and makes it impossible to avoid the ones that don't. And looking in the cancer mirror shows you the places where you're not quite what you could be.

For me, again and again, the cancer mirror has shown the same shadowed place: being able to admit that I'm not OK is something that I find difficult. My 'Be Perfect' driver means I don't want to worry people, and I don't want to feel that I'm letting them down.

I think that this is partly because my way of coping with cancer has always been to focus on the positives, so I don't always see that I am struggling. Maybe I'm afraid that if I once allow myself to not be doing well, I will turn into a wibbling mass of self pity and never be able to take on human form again, with my family and friends taking it in turns to push me around in a wheelbarrow. But a couple of conversations have made me think recently. One was when Alan – yes, my husband Alan, who I spend time with every day and who I think that I talk to about everything – told me that he had only realised when he read the blog that I wasn't feeling 100 per cent. The other was talking to Gerri, who came with me for the PICC insertion, and who said she was sorry that I opted to be home alone afterwards when she and Nathalie would have loved to look after me and it would have been OK to let them do so.

So. I am trying to learn.

There's really one message I'm trying to get over in this whole chapter: *Please, don't try to do cancer on your own.*

BAH! THINKING 🐉

A visualization for when someone you love is dancing with cancer

Sit somewhere comfortable where you won't be disturbed. Take some time to think about your loved one. Don't think about them now: think about them before cancer, happy and well. Fix a picture of your well, happy loved one in your mind.

Radiotherapy: It's me again!

HOW RADIOTHERAPY WORKS

Cancer treatment, in essence, is a three-pronged approach: slash, poison and burn. Surgery slashes the cancer out, while chemotherapy works on the principle that there could be cancer cells anywhere in the body and so poisoning them from within is the best approach. Radiotherapy, for its part, focuses on the problem area and burns it from without.

And that's 'burn' as in nuke, as in fire radioactivity at it. Obviously, this is dangerous. The blackly funny thing about both chemotherapy and radiotherapy is that one of the side effects can be – wait for it – cancer. I know. You couldn't make it up.

Radiotherapy is used in many ways. It can be used to try to shrink or destroy a cancer altogether, or to shrink it before surgery. It can be used as a bit of extra insurance when a tumour appears to have been removed. It can be used to reduce pain as part of palliative care.

Radiotherapy can be given externally or internally. Internal radiotherapy is a treatment for some bone, blood and thyroid cancers, and works by introducing radioactivity directly into the body, either via implants or liquids. (Isotope milkshake, anyone? No, I didn't think so.)

The (more common) external sort of radiotherapy involves having X-ray-type beams fired at specific areas of the body, repeatedly for a given period of time. Each dose (or 'fraction') destroys the cells in its path. But the point of this treatment is to make sure the cells are really, properly dead. And so another dose, soon afterwards – usually the next day – is given. So any cells staggering back to life get zapped again. I imagined the cells of my breast like a crowd of people crammed into a park, then the wrecking ball of radiotherapy plunging through them, knocking them all over. Undeterred, they get up again, but before they can get fully upright, the ball strikes again, knocking them flying. Again the cell-people rise ... but a little slower. Wham! comes the ball. Eventually – after, say, 20 times – the cell-people in the park stop getting up. So if there are any cancer-cell-people, the wrecking ball has got rid of them. But there's a lot of collateral damage: all of those perfectly innocent cell-people are going to take a while to recover.

However radiotherapy comes, it is designed to act directly on the area where the cancer is/might be.

GETTING READY

Radiotherapy units need to be built in underground areas (but really, it's very safe), so not all hospitals have one. My main treatment hospital, St George's in Tooting, didn't, so I opted to go to the Royal Marsden in Kensington instead. Some time before my chemotherapy finished, I went for a planning visit. I was quite excited about being treated at the Marsden, because it has an excellent reputation, and arriving there was thrilling because there were things like an absence of hospital smell, real live fish in a fish tank not green with slime, and magazines that were less than a year old. Oh, and the chairs weren't screwed down.

There was the usual taking-of-the-medical-history ('only a tonsillectomy') and this was the occasion on which I was asked, without irony, the rather fantastic question, 'Apart from the cancer, are you in good health?' (This was at the zenith of chemotherapy side effects. I had had to take the lift to the basement rather than walk down one flight of stairs. Yes, one. Yes, down. I believe my answer was a hollow laughter-like sound and an eye roll.) The procedure was explained. My treatment would be scheduled; I would be given an appointment to come in for measurements and to meet my team and be shown the machine. Someone may have drawn on me, or maybe that was later.

I explained my position: that I was self-employed, that I couldn't afford not to work for a month – this wasn't strictly true, financially at least, but emotionally and psychologically it was right on the money – that I wasn't sure that the treatment was strictly necessary and that I would appreciate a bit of flexibility. We compared diaries and found a stretch of time where I was only going to be away for two days and either not working or working in London for the rest of the time. Radiotherapy was duly scheduled.

The second planning visit – in the week before radiotherapy was due to begin – was a bit more hands-on. Hands, pens, needles. My medical history was taken ('Only a tonsillectomy. And cancer'). Then I changed into a gown and waited in a side room while the patient before me had a panic attack when going through the process of having measurements taken. I listened while trying not to, and my heart ached. I thanked whatever it is that should be thanked for my absence of claustrophobia, hospital-phobia and needle-phobia (most of the time, at least), and I knitted at a sock and waited, while the technicians came and apologized for the delay every ten minutes or so.

It was my turn eventually: I was escorted into the room where a vast cyclops of a radiotherapy machine waited. Below the great eye was a bench, and I lay down on it as instructed and shuffled my backside to the assigned backside area. (Helpfully, there was a little backside shelf. They think of everything.) I was asked to raise my right arm above my head, the bench moved up to the correct position, and then the Arranging of the Breast began.

Because radiotherapy is so dangerous – although you'll never hear that word used in a radiotherapy unit, where 'powerful' is the adjective of choice – it's important that the X-ray beam is targeted as accurately as possible on the treatment area and shouldn't stray anywhere else. In my case, I was having 15 days of irradiation of the whole of my right breast, plus a five-day 'booster' treatment focusing only on the area where the cancer had been. The trick for breast cancer patients is getting the radiotherapy through the breast without it touching the chest wall, which could be ~~dangerous~~ powerful. The other trick is trying to get a part of the body that is entirely muscle-free – and is usually contained by a DD cup – to get into the correct position and stay there. Eventually the team managed it. Then they drew on me, wrote down the co-ordinates, and then made two tiny tattoos, one between my breasts and one on my right side, to help them to line the radiotherapy beam up.

(Like never being able to have blood taken from my right arm again, this incidental side effect bugs me more than it, perhaps, should. From time to time I think about getting the tiny blue dot between my breasts converted into a tiny blue tattoo. But I've had enough of needles for now.)

I left feeling as though I had been in good hands. (No pun intended.) The Marsden seemed professional and, well, a little bit slick, which, compared to St George's shambolic, short-staffed, can't-find-notes approach, was rather refreshing. … to start with.

BAH! THINKING

A meditation for preparing for radiotherapy

Get comfortable. Breathe slowly and calmly, and think only about your breath, until it feels as though your breath is breathing you.

Now think about the place in your body that is going to be irradiated. Think about how strong the healthy cells are. Think about how well they are going to cope. Feel proud of your body, so strong and so able in spite of all. Imagine that part of your body bathed in cool, clean light.

When you are ready, open your eyes.

Practise this every day, until it becomes second nature; then you can do it on the way to the hospital and in the waiting room.

TREATMENT

Here's how it goes:

- Arrive: 10–20 minutes before appointment: sign in with reception. Every day, have this conversation:

S: I'm here to sign in.

Receptionist: Hello, Mrs Butland.

S: Hello. Please, call me Stephanie.

Receptionist: Stephanie. Right-o.

Except on the last day, which went:

S: I'm here to sign in.

Receptionist: Hello, Mrs Butland.

S: (defeated) Hello.

- Wait: Anything from 0–40 minutes (depending on whether I'm just after the man who has panic attacks or not).

- Be called: Get shown into therapy area and change into a gown behind a curtain.

- Be arranged: After the minimum of 'How are you today?' chat, get onto the bench. Those co-ordinates from the planning visit are then projected onto the wall, the lights go down, and two light beams are projected onto me. They must cross in exactly the right place, so I try not to mind while I am twisted and hauled into position. (Early on I am told in no uncertain terms that my attempts to help, by moving my body myself, are not helpful. A bit like moving your own fingers during a manicure.)

- Be left: Even though everyone is quite sure that the risks of radiotherapy are minimal, everyone who isn't me runs behind a big thick wall before starting the treatment. Thoughtfully, the tiles directly above the machine have been replaced with a transparent panel with palm tree fronds and blue sky to gaze upon. This amuses me for the 90 seconds or so my treatment takes.

- Be treated: The machine whirrs and buzzes. There's a rat-a-tat sound, too, which I fondly imagine is a Geiger counter, although I never think to ask. After 30 seconds, the machine lugubriously whirrs round so that it is irradiating my breast from the opposite side. Another 30 seconds, and I am done for the day.

- Be dismissed: The technicians return, the bed is lowered, then it's back behind the curtain, dressed and up the stairs, blinking in the late spring light.

- Repeat: x20.

SUNDAY, 17 MAY 2009 [ABRIDGED]: WEEK 1 REVIEW

Well, it's a week since I started the radiotherapy regime: five days on, two days off. (The powers that be insist that this is a careful balance of treatment v rest, perfectly calculated for optimum effectiveness. Hmmmm. Methinks that if this were true – and the 'weekends off' thing therefore a happy coincidence – I'd be having treatment on the Bank Holiday Monday, which strangely, I'm not. Odd, *non*?)

Anyway. A mixed week, I think.

On the positive side, radiotherapy is neither painful nor stressful. No needles, tablets or particular indignities – at least, if you don't mind having your breasts exposed on a regular basis. I'm pretty used to it. (Since being diagnosed with breast cancer, I mean. I don't have a former career as a topless model, pole dancer or similar.)

[...]

On the negative side, a two-and-a-half hour chunk out of each day is a bore, and my breast is pink and a little bit sore – as though I'd left it (but not the rest of my body) out in the sun too long. I've had to start wearing non-underwired bras, which doesn't give my 36DD assets quite the boost they're used to. (I should add 'vanity' as a label for posts. Or maybe we could just take vanity as read....) My tattoos seem to slip out of alignment between the first and second blasts of radiation, which means being rearranged – not a problem, I'm assured, but it would all be quicker and easier if they didn't. Trying to get myself to the unit on the days I'm working is a bit of an issue (the department operates on a strict 9-5 schedule, as do most of my training days – you can see the difficulty). Oh, and the Fabled Radiotherapy Tiredness hit me like a truck carrying a load of cement yesterday afternoon. 2.30pm to 5.30pm is a complete blank.

Still … I think, on balance, the positives outweigh the negatives, so far. There's another really nice thing about this stage of treatment too, which I hadn't anticipated. It's the people in the waiting room.

Pre- and post-surgery, waiting rooms are full of people blank-eyed with disbelief or pain. There's quite a lot of quiet crying. Waiting for chemotherapy, people are kind to each other, and chat, and admire hats/scarves/wigs, but beneath it all there's a grimness, a fear, while they wait to have their names called and get back onto the cancer dancefloor for another three weeks of varying degrees of unpleasantness.

But waiting for radiotherapy is another experience altogether. People do chat, and laugh, without covering their mouths and looking guilty. People read the newspapers and comment on the news. They admire each other's hair and compare notes on regrowth rates. Maybe they knit (OK, that was me) or crochet (that wasn't). They bring friends and family to keep them company, and talk to them about normal, everyday stuff, like what to do at the weekend and when their daughter's baby is due. I guess there's a bit of demob-happiness around. Of course, radiotherapy doesn't mean that the dance with cancer is truly over. But for many people, it means a kind of normality is in sight. Me included. One week down, three to go.

BAH! THINKING 🐉

Coping with the process

I found it best to be what I thought of as 'mentally absent' while I was being arranged and irradiated.

1. Work your way through the alphabet, thinking of the name of someone you know for each letter. When you're done, do the same thing again, but with surnames this time.

2. Choose a four-digit number at random (say, 7603) and a number between 1 and 10 (say, 7) and then count down from the big number in increments of the small number (7603, 7596, 7989 ...)

3. Decide what to have for dinner.

4. Try to remember everything you did yesterday.

5. Think about whose birthday is coming up next and plan what to give them.

6. Put together a fantasy dinner party, a fantasy cabinet, or a fantasy football team.

7. See how many jokes you can remember.

8. Think about the last book you read.

9. Imagine what each of your loved ones is doing right now.

10. Plan something nice to be doing this time next month.

SIDE EFFECTS

What happens during radiotherapy is the equivalent of leaving your breast out in tropical sun every day. So the main side effect was, more or less, severe sunburn.

My skin turned red and got itchy. (It still is a little bit suntanned-looking. I don't think that will ever fully go away.) My nipple got a bit peely and itched. My breast hurt when I rolled onto it as I slept.

All of these side effects were greatly helped by slathering my breast in pure aloe vera gel morning and night. I kept the gel in the fridge and putting it on was heavenly.

There's also the Fabled Radiotherapy Tiredness, which I was warned about again and again. The theory is that the body is making furious and increasingly hysterical efforts to get those cells in the cell-park standing up before the wrecking ball comes through again, and this takes lots of energy. Although the tiredness did get me in the end – the kind of weariness that starts in your soul and gradually eats through all of you – I'm not completely convinced it was the radiotherapy that did it. I think it was more likely to have been the boredom, the 90-minute daily round trip, the fact that every day I was being reminded that I had had a cancer. (At least with chemotherapy there are whole groups of days when you don't have to have anything to do with a hospital.) There was all of that thinking time, all of that schlepping up and down roads that became tediously familiar. For someone who is not a big one for routine anyway – I've only twice had proper 9-5 jobs and I didn't like them either time – this really didn't suit.

TUESDAY, 26 MAY 2009 [ABRIDGED]: WEEK 2 REVIEW

So, last week saw another 5 radiotherapy treatments come and go, with very little variation in the routine or the symptoms. Last Monday and Tuesday I was working, so finished training at 4.30pm (my delegates very graciously agreed to a shortened lunchtime to accommodate this), got into a cab, and travelled breathlessly across to the Royal Marsden where I was treated in the final time slot of the day. (Actually, I think they invented a final time slot just for me.) The rest of the week was more low key, and I pottered at home, went to the gym, saw friends, and went for treatment. By Friday I really was shattered, but it is a different kind of tiredness, this Fabled Radiotherapy Tiredness. It's somewhere between jet lag and a mild hangover, but without the foreign trip or the wine…. which makes it a tad tedious. I found last week that I wasn't sleeping very well either – I think I was rolling onto my tender breast (not tender in the Mills and Boon sense, tender in an 'Ow! Don't press there!' kind of a way) and waking myself up. I took sleeping pills on a couple of nights which helped me to catch up with my sleep a bit, and thus rejoin the human race. (As anyone who knows me will tell you, a Stephanie who has not been sleeping well is a thing to be avoided at all costs.)

Alan and I went out to play on Friday night, took it easy on Saturday, took it very easy on Sunday, and went out to play again yesterday. So I'm feeling quite recharged, although weepiness set in over lunch yesterday. Would anyone who was in Le Pain Quotidien on the South Bank please note that my husband is a wonderful, kind and considerate man, who did not make me cry. (I always feel bad for Alan when I cry in public, as I assume people assume that he has upset me. Which tells you quite a lot of the assumptions I make, I guess.) I had a moment of feeling utterly overwhelmed by this dance with cancer; the nearer I get to the end of treatment, the more inclined I am to look back, and the whole thing seems bigger and scarier in retrospect than it was at the time I was going through it.

I'm still sporting a slightly pink, slightly swollen breast, but it's not getting any worse, and I am encouraged by the thought that I'm more than half way through the radiotherapy treatments now […], although not halfway through the timeline – work intervenes next week, which I'm glad about. (A bit of normal now and then does wonders.) Once it's all over I will look forward to binning my un-underwired bras and getting a bit of uplift going again. Once the Fabled Radiotherapy Tiredness is over, I'm hoping for a bit of uplift in life in general too!

THE GOOD RADIOTHERAPY PATIENT VERSUS ME

The good radiotherapy patient clears her diary and does exactly what she's told. I scheduled work and had to have the occasional day rescheduled. This earned me plenty of chats about Taking Treatment Seriously, and a couple of massive taxi fares as I hared in from the other side of London to make sure I got to the hospital in time.

The good radiotherapy patient is given her next day's appointment when she is at the hospital. I insisted on having my schedule of appointments in advance so I could plan round them. This perplexed the staff who – like, I think, many people who haven't had cancer but think they know what they would do if they did – could not seem to imagine why anyone who was having cancer treatment would be doing anything except have cancer treatment. So if I said something like, 'Could I please have an early or late appointment next Monday because I'm going shopping for the day?' my request would often be met with a raised eyebrow (subtext: you think you are but when it comes to it you will be Too Tired) or a hearty, 'Good for you!' type comment (subtext: you brave little soldier, shopping and behaving like a normal person in the face of cancer).

The good radiotherapy patient doesn't ask questions. I asked things like, 'If it's so critical that I have treatment every day, why isn't the unit open on weekends or Bank Holiday

Monday?' and 'Why are you allowed to miss a day a week but I'm not?'

The good radiotherapy patient is happy to be alive and considers any alteration to her lifestyle a price worth paying for that. I fiercely resented having to put away my underwire bras for a month and wear the non-wired sort. They gave me, as Joy put it, 'breasts like a grandma,' they meant that none of my clothes hung right, and as I'd already gained weight from chemotherapy they didn't do anything to make me feel any less a fat frump.

The good radiotherapy patient speaks when spoken to and is as inconspicuous as possible. I spent a couple of weeks trying to build a rapport with the people I was treated by, a serious bunch possibly a little inclined to take themselves a little too seriously. I got a little way with Rachel but realized I was simply annoying everyone else. I stopped.

The good radiotherapy patient accepts that not everything always goes to plan, and is prepared to come in late or early or on a Saturday when a machine breaks down. I was a good radiotherapy patient in that respect at least.

MONDAY, 1 JUNE 2009: END OF PART 1

When I finished training today I got straight into a cab (well, I left the venue first, I wasn't training in the street) and headed off to the Royal Marsden. I was on a 5pm deadline and if I didn't make it I would 'compromise my entire course of treatment.'

(Strangely, this did not apply to last Monday, which was a Bank Holiday. You gotta love the NHS.)

The taxi driver was well intentioned…. when I told him where I was going he clocked my hair, immediately turned off his radio and drove me through central London in complete silence. I can only presume that this was out of respect for my imminent demise. (He drove as though my life depended on it. In some lights, I suppose he was right.)

So, thanks to my ambulance/taxi driver, I arrived with a good couple of minutes to spare… and wasn't seen til 5.20, not that I minded. And then I underwent number 15 of 15 radiotherapy treatments to the whole of my right breast. I have 4 'boost' treatments – only to the area where the cancer was – next week, but the general radiation is now over.

(If you can hear a squeaky little voice shouting a faint 'hurrah!'; you're not imagining things. It's my very toasty nipple talking. Boy, is it sore.)

So… there goes another part of my dance with cancer. Compared to surgery and chemotherapy, it was physically easier, but there is something quite draining about doing the same thing every (week)day for three weeks. (I realise that all of you with proper jobs are now saying 'Chuh! Tell me about it, sunshine,' but bear in mind that my entire life is organised around my low boredom threshold.) There's been no escape from cancer these last three weeks; I haven't been able to play at being a normal person – not that cancer makes me abnormal, but you know what I mean. But on the up side, I've been nurtured and checked on and in an environment with a lot of people who are In The Same Boat. I think, once next week is over, I might miss that a little bit. Daft, eh?

WHAT I REMEMBER ABOUT RADIOTHERAPY

- I remember the way we patients smiled at each other every day. It was a 'We're surviving this! It's nearly over!' smile rather than the grim, shocked, 'Isn't this awful? How can it be happening?' almost-smiles of the chemotherapy unit.

- I remember some people – I'm assuming they were the palliative care patients – being wheeled down from the main hospital for their treatments. There were no smiles then. They were barely conscious. Barely alive, even.

- I remember leaving the unit late one evening – I had been working and was the last patient – and seeing one of the technicians wheeling a trolley full of the rubber masks used for patients with mouth and throat cancers. The masks are made to help keep the head in the right position and target the radiotherapy. This means that these poor souls must keep their mouths wide open for the duration of treatment. And it meant that the trolley was full of rubber heads with blank eyes and wide, screaming maws. I can still see them now.

- I remember gradually falling out of love with the Marsden and forgiving St George's some of its failings. St George's was scruffy and tatty and disorganized, but the Marsden was smug and very pleased with itself. I later told one of the nurses who'd had some training at the Marsden about that feeling. She nodded her agreement. 'They have what they call The Marsden Way,' she said. 'It's a bit much.'

BAH! THINKING
Managing radiotherapy time

You might be lucky. You might live next door to a radiotherapy unit. If you don't, chances are you're looking at a round-trip every day for a month or so. So it's Green Hat thinking time again: here are some things you could do to escape the feeling that you are doing nothing but going back and forwards to be nuked every day:

- Have a book by an author you enjoy, and read it only on the way to and from the hospital; no matter how exciting it gets, wait until your next day's journey to read some more.

- Find out who lives/works near the hospital and combine radiotherapy with seeing them. Diane lived and Jude worked in Fulham near the Marsden, so we would meet for lunch or coffee before or after my appointment.

- Think about having some additional therapy that will heal you in a more gentle way. Once a week I'd go and have a treatment at Breast Cancer Haven, conveniently close to the Marsden. This charity provides 20 hours of complementary (and complimentary!) therapies to anyone with breast cancer. So I'd have a massage, or a session of therapy or counselling.

- Arrive early and have lunch somewhere lovely while you read your radiotherapy-only book.

- Wonder about the people who live in the houses you pass on the way to the hospital.

- Take someone with you.

- Walk there. I challenged myself to walk parts of the journey, as I tried to teach myself to start moving, and breathing, and functioning normally again.

- Knit. (Of course.)

HOW TO HELP: Things to do for the radiotherapy patient in your life

1. Source some all-natural, additive-free aloe vera gel and some unperfumed shower gel for your loved one. Tiny particles of metal in perfumed soaps and cosmetics can stay on the skin and react with the radiotherapy beams, making reactions worse.

2. And something very luxurious and lovely-smelling for when it's all over.

3. Find out where the radiotherapy unit is and think about what's nearby. Suggest combining radiotherapy with a trip to one of those nearby places.

4. Offer to come along. But only if you're OK with hospitals. Being accompanied by someone who is doing their best to freak out in an unobtrusive way in order to not upset you is actually quite stressful.

5. Here's another one of those annoying conversations to avoid:

Friend/colleague: So, where are you with your treatment now?

Me: I'm having radiotherapy now.

Friend/colleague: Radiotherapy. So that's ...?

Me: I'm going to the Marsden every day for a month, to get my breast irradiated in case there are any cancer cells left. There aren't, obviously.

Friend/colleague: No, of course not. Does it hurt?

Me: No, not really. It's a bit like sunburn. And really boring. I have to go every day and it's an hour-and-a-half round-trip.

Friend/colleague: Oh, well. At least it's not as bad as chemotherapy.

That last sentence. Right there. No, it's not as bad as chemotherapy. But, frankly, few things are. You wouldn't (I hope) say, 'Your mother's died? I'm so sorry. Still, at least it wasn't your wife.' If you fell out of a tree and broke lots of bits of you, I can't imagine you'd be glad to hear the paramedics remark, 'Hey, this is nowhere near as bad as falling off the roof of a block of flats.'

Just because it isn't chemotherapy doesn't mean it isn't anything. It's a painful, time-consuming treatment that reminds you every day that you are dancing with cancer. It itches and burns. It's undignified. It's tiring. Respect that. Try:

Me: No, not really. It's a bit like sunburn. And really boring.

Friend/colleague: Sunburn isn't any fun. Would you like me to come with you one day?

Or:

Me: No, not really. It's a bit like sunburn. And really boring.

Friend/colleague: When will it be done with? We should do something to celebrate.

Or even:

Me: No, not really. It's a bit like sunburn. And really boring.

Friend/colleague: It's still treatment and it can't be easy for you. Can I come and keep you company sometime?

THE END

My last day of radiotherapy was a Friday. I had a breast as bright as a robin's and was thoroughly fed up with the whole thing. But, it was the last day, and Alan and I were meeting friends for dinner that evening, and so I put on something that looked reasonable with the grandma-bra and off I went. As I got dressed after the treatment, one of the technicians said, 'So this is your last one?' I agreed that it was. 'Well, good luck,' he said. And that was it. No balloons, no party-poppers, not even a round of applause. I walked up the stairs out of the basement and into the light. (Into the daylight, that is. The basement wasn't in darkness. But there was something oppressive about it: you knew you were underground.) Alan was there to meet me, and I had a little cry, right there on a pavement in Kensington, with his arms tight around me, while the number 14 buses and the taxis thundered by. I'd like to say I felt lucky, but really I just felt tired.

Drug trial: The amazing exploding head

WHY THE DRUGS?

The medical profession is nothing if not thorough when it comes to cancer. We're talking a belt, braces, piece of twine, buttons and velcro approach. It goes something like this:

1. Surgery removes the cancer.

   • But in case it hasn't ...

2. Chemotherapy kills cancer cells from within the body's systems.

   • But in case it doesn't ...

3. Radiotherapy nukes the area with the cancer and destroys the cells there over and over, until nothing lives.

   • But in case something does live ...

4. Drug therapy deprives it of what it feeds on, so it cannot grow.

   • But in case it does grow ...

5. Off you go, back down the snake to surgery. (If you're lucky.)

When cancers are removed from the body, they are analysed and categorized. I had accidentally grown a HER2-positive, oestrogen-positive cancer. If the HER2 or oestrogen had 'negative' after them, that would have been good news, because it would have meant that the cancer that had been growing in my breast had been doodling about on its own, a bit like those lone protestors you see in tents covered in pictures outside Downing Street. That 'positive' makes it a bit more of a force to be reckoned with: a bit more of an anti-nuclear protest march in 1984.

So, let's start with HER2. No, I'd never heard of it either. HER2 is a receptor which is found on the outside of some cancer cells, and its presence allows the cancer to utilize a substance which occurs naturally in the body, called human epidermal growth factor. Now, you don't want a growth factor hooking up with a cancer cell. Oh no. It's like chucking a bucket of water over a gremlin. Really not a good idea, because the cancer can use the growth factor to help its cells to divide fast, fast, fast.

A similar thing happens with oestrogen: oestrogen-positive cancers utilize the body's hormones to accelerate their growth.

So drugs have been developed to stop the body's uptake of HER2 and of oestrogen, to starve any stray cancer cells out.

TREATING HER2+ CANCER WITH HERCEPTIN

Herceptin (or trastuzumab, to give it its Sunday name) represented a massive breakthrough in cancer treatment when it was first developed, because it was the first drug able to effectively block HER2 receptors, so that the growth factor can no longer feed the cancer cell. Simple, yet effective – the pharmaceutical equivalent of locking your door from the inside and leaving the key in it.

Clinical trials of herceptin showed it to be fabulous at preventing a return of breast cancer, and a year of herceptin treatment quickly became the standard of care in the UK. However, research into the effectiveness of the drug continues. Put baldly, at the time of writing we know it works, but we don't know how it works best, so trials are going on looking at the duration of treatment, the stages of cancer it is given at, and whether it should be given at the same time as or after chemotherapy.

Herceptin also has some drawbacks. It's expensive: a year's supply of the drug costs around £50,000. And it has to be given intravenously, every three weeks, a process that takes a couple of hours. It has some potentially serious side effects, heart failure being top of the list. It causes what oncologists and nurses blithely refer to as 'mild flu-like symptoms', which sound like nothing much until you find yourself aching so much you can barely get out of bed, and with nostrils so dry and painful that your nose bleeds pretty much constantly. So – and this is probably not just owing to the sore noses out there – researchers are already looking for the next thing, the better thing, the thing that makes us all talk about herceptin the way we now talk about legwarmers, conveniently forgetting how for a good few years back there in the 1980s we wouldn't have been seen dead without them.

THE ALLTO TRIAL

So, I was not offered herceptin. I was offered a place on the ALLTO trial, which was looking at another existing cancer drug, lapatinib, proven to be fiercely effective in treating late-stage cancers. (That last bit, sadly, is medical speak for 'keeps you alive a bit longer'.) The ALLTO trial, a global trial, was looking at the efficacy of a year of herceptin versus a year of lapatinib versus a year of simultaneous herceptin and lapatinib versus a year of herceptin followed by lapatinib versus a year of herceptin and lapatinib given as jelly shaped like a rabbit (probably).

I was excited to take part in the trial, partly because I like feeling that I am Helping, but mainly because lapatinib comes in tablet form. So if I got onto that arm of the trial I would be spared the ritual of needles, tubes and half a day in a hospital every three weeks. The side effects, I was told, would be much the same, whichever arm of the trial I was allocated. But it seemed to me that taking tablets every day would be a step toward normality. Lots of people take tablets. Taking tablets is a pretty average activity, I reasoned, whether for blood pressure or contraception or constipation or because you think starflower oil is helping you to be a bit less moody. So even if I was taking tablets for a scary reason – to starve those last dogged cancer cells into submission – I would also be taking a step away from being a patient. And I wouldn't have to go back to the place where I sat having chemotherapy drugs pushed and pumped into my unwilling veins.

I crossed my fingers.

BAH! THINKING
Getting on drug trials

If you are asked to take part in a drug trial there is strict guidance about the information that must be given to you. It's pretty good. But here are some other questions you might want to ask.

1. Have other patients you have treated been on this trial? What has happened to them?

2. Why have you suggested that I take part in this trial?

3. Are there other drug trials coming up that I would be eligible for, that this trial would preclude me from taking part in?

4. How might side effects differ from the standard treatment?

5. What are the implications of taking part in this trial for my long-term health?

6. What's the worst that could happen?

TAKING PART IN A DRUG TRIAL

Drug trials are serious, proper, rigorous things. I imagined it would be something like:

1. Pick a card, any card.

2. Take drugs as instructed on card.

3. Let us know if/when you have another cancer.

4. Get someone to let us know if/when you die and what kills you.

It turned out to be a bit more involved.

First, there was the sheaf of papers I was given to read about the trial. I scanned through it, asked my mum about the drugs and how they worked (she was a pharmacy technician for many years and can tell you what everything does without blinking), made sure none of the likely side effects was weight gain, and decided to go ahead.

Next time I was at the hospital the oncologist took me through the details and possible side effects of the trial. She told me that the cancer that had been removed from my breast would be sent to Milan, where the ALLTO team would retest it and confirm that it was HER2+. (Sadly, I was not allowed to escort it.) And then it was over to the drug trial nurse to arrange the tests and fill in the forms.

If there were a scale of drug potency – and there probably is somewhere – then the kind of drugs I was going to be given would be way up at the end that isn't paracetamol. Owing to that, the side effects can be extremely damaging to the body – particularly the heart and lungs – so tests were needed to make sure that I was fit enough to take part in the trial, and to establish a base position so that the impact of the drugs could be monitored over the year. The tests would be repeated at three-month intervals during the trial, and every year for five years once my year of treatment was over.

First, blood was taken. Lots and lots of tubes of blood. (The PICC line did make this delightfully straightforward, not least because the usual 'take-a-ticket-and-wait-a-week-until-your-number-is-called' phlebotomists don't do PICC lines so it was done on the ward, without a wait.) Then I was sent for an ECG and echocardiogram. The ECG measures the heart's activity, so lots of stickers were stuck around my shoulders, chest and back, clips attached to them, and a machine churned out lines of peaks and troughs which I took to signify that I was alive and ... well, let's just stick with alive. The echocardiogram is an ultrasound scan of the heart – I stopped myself from asking 'Is it a girl or a boy?' because I imagine everyone does, but it was very, very tempting – which looks closely at how the valves are operating, what volume of blood is being pushed through, and generally gives a good overall picture of heart health. Finally, I had a CT scan. CT (computerized tomography) scans create a very detailed sort of three-dimensional X-ray of what's going on inside the body. Because the inside of the lungs are filled with so many tiny pathways, the scanner needs a little help in seeing clearly, so something nasty needs to be pushed through the bloodstream at high volume for the duration of the scan (about ten seconds). This meant getting a line in. No problem! I said, waving my PICC line around. The PICC line, however, couldn't be used; something to do with valves and volume and pressure. There was much sighing and shaking of heads over my hopeless veins, and the technician decided he wasn't even going to try to get a line in, but would get a doctor to do it. The doctor took the 'just ram it in and hope for the best' approach, which actually worked. I was asked to keep my fingers on the vein: I'd feel it bulge, and if it became too painful or felt as though it might burst, I was to shout. The technician told me how safe the procedure was by running off behind a big thick wall and talking to me via intercom. The machine talked to me, which was a bit disquieting, telling me to breathe in, hold my breath, breathe out. My vein bulged but didn't burst. It hurt, but just a little.

swallow them straight away they left a taste in my mouth that lingered longer than raw garlic.

But I didn't mind. Not really. Every morning, as I stood by the kitchen sink and swallowed the orange monsters one by one, I thought about how glad I was to be taking tablets and not heading for hospital. I added up how many days (nine, at least) and how many cannulations (18, at least, but that was if they all went really, really well, which was unlikely) I was avoiding.

When the diarrhoea began I was a little less enthused, but still cheerful. It didn't come with pain and I didn't have to remain within 25 metres of a loo at all times: 'manageable' was the word I think I used when I told Kay about it. (When you are on a drug trial there are protocols for everything so you can't go treating your own symptoms with over-the-counter meds. Oh no. You tell the drug trial nurse, who looks up the protocols, consults with ALLTO central, takes advice from them about appropriate treatment, and then tells you what to do. Which, in this case, was to take over-the-counter diarrhoea medication. Well, better safe than sorry.)

Then I woke up one Sunday morning with a face swollen beyond all recognition. And I mean beyond all recognition. I posted a picture on my blog and my mother rang me up to say she wouldn't have known me. When your own mother doesn't know you ... that, my friend, is unrecognizable. I'd gone to bed with a bit of a rash the night before, but had put it down to being out in the sun all day. But that morning saw my skin mottled and stretched, my eyes disappearing as my cheeks and eyelids swelled. Alan's face told me it was every bit as bad as I thought it was. I was almost afraid to let the children see me, although they were mature beyond their years when confronted with a mother who looked more like an exercise in CGI. Elsewhere on my body, I had swelling and rashes. I wanted to scratch but didn't dare. I was moon-faced and afraid.

We called the hospital and then headed on down. I was seen pretty quickly: bloods, cannulation, and going through what exactly had happened with the on-call oncologist (who was delightful. Not 'delightful-for-an-oncologist' ... properly delightful). She had to go off and read all of the drug trial protocols and consult ALLTO central, of course, but she kept us informed of what was going on. Her hypothesis (later trashed by my usual oncologist, but it made sense to me) was that the trial drug blocked not only HER2 but also HER1, and the side effects I was suffering were due to my body being starved of HER1.

The treatment was intravenous steroids and anti-histamines, and crossed fingers. After a few hours we were given oral antihistamine and sent home. I remember that evening: we all sat around trying to convince ourselves that the swelling was going down. I went to bed, and I slept for a while, but I woke at 2 a.m. with my skin feeling stretched to breaking point. My vision was limited to a slit because my cheeks were swollen so much. My skin had the texture of parmesan cheese. I got up and looked in the mirror. Big mistake. I woke Alan, we called the hospital, and I was instructed to come down straight away. We decided that I would go on my own; it was quicker and more efficient than waking the children or finding someone to come and stay with them.

I called a taxi and was glad of the dark. Sitting in the A&E waiting room – which, mercifully, I didn't have to do for long

– gave me food for thought. I knew I looked strange; what I didn't know was how looking strange changed the way the world looks at you. People did double-takes or made a point of avoiding looking at my face. There was no malice, just the brain's need to look twice at what it doesn't understand, or the protection of avoiding what is uncomfortable. All perfectly understandable. All a bit of a shock to someone who can usually get a seat on a crowded train with a well-aimed smile.

I was soon in a consulting room on A&E, where the first thing to do was to get a line into my shattered, parched veins. Three or four people had a go. Every time someone came into the room they would ask me the same questions:

Is the swelling getting worse?

Does your throat feel tight?

Are you able to breathe OK?

Given that none of my face was where it ought to be, I was pretty disorientated, so I couldn't really tell. But the more I was asked, the more I began to wonder. My body was tense and tired from the repeated attempts to get a needle into a vein. It seemed that the people treating me couldn't get away from my swollen features fast enough. Eventually, the nurses gave up with the needles, and decided to fetch the doctor on duty. I was told to shout if I felt my throat get tighter.

It was 3 a.m. I was in a bare, bright room, barely able to see, hot and itchy and utterly unprepared for this unexpected adventure into the world of circus freakery. My breathing seemed short and the speed with which I was seen was enough to frighten me: I'd barely had time to sit down before I was ushered through. I had never seriously entertained the notion that breast cancer would kill me; but at that moment, alone and swollen, I thought that this drug might. I remember lying on a trolley in a hospital gown that was frayed and faded, elastoplasts and gauze covering the needle-pricks in my usable arm, so much cheek I couldn't see down and so much chin I could barely move my head, and I thought: I could die here. If my throat is swelling, if my veins won't play, I could suffocate in this place, now, tonight.

Everything seemed to stop. It was as though I'd gone to visit The Museum of Stephanie and had come across a room in which there was a single exhibit, probably made of marble, probably a mixture of icy curves and jagged corners, called 'The moment at which Stephanie thinks she might die, quite soon.' I walked round and round the sculpture, looking at it from all sides, and I had two thoughts:

- I've survived cancer. I'm damned if I'm dying of a horse pill, and looking like this.

- If I do die tonight, it won't be the end of the world. It will be, for a while, of course, but my children are intelligent and resourceful and strong, my husband and I have stored up more happy memories in the 12 years we've known each other than some people manage in a lifetime, and my parents and friends will understand that I did everything I could to stay. I've done much and regret little. I could have done more, but hey, I'd probably still think that if I died in my preferred setting: age 93, lying in a hammock in a red swimsuit, somewhere Mediterranean, glass of champagne to hand, great book just finished, friends and family nearby.

The door banged open and the doctor strode in. He took one look at my arm, said 'No problem!' and what he did next felt as though he'd backed 100 metres out of the room so as to get a good run at it and then rammed the needle in at high speed. I didn't half squeal. But it was done. Steroids and antibiotics happened, fast.

I don't remember being taken to a ward, but I was: it was a sort of holding ward for people admitted overnight. There was noise and crying and shouting for nurses. I stayed in my bed and kept the curtains drawn, profoundly embarrassed by my face, thoroughly fed up with the whole thing. I rang Alan as soon as I felt I could do so without disturbing anyone else, and told him I was OK, but I wasn't, not really. I had a little cry, but my tears stung my raw skin. I tried to sleep, but nothing was comfortable. As soon as I dozed off someone would wake me to give me tea/breakfast/drugs or ask if I could breathe.

I was amazed by how quickly the drugs started to work. By lunchtime the scorched, stretched feeling was receding and I could see most of the world and move my head comfortably. The on-call oncologist had told me to expect a visit from my usual oncologist after clinic that morning, and sure enough she duly arrived, with her intern and her lunch freshly bought from Marks and Spencer in a bag.

There are many words I could use to describe my oncologist, but two that wouldn't even make the reserve list would be 'emotional' and 'intelligent'. Oh no. Picture the scene: I have been through a sad and scary night. Just when I thought my dance with cancer was drawing to a close, a fresh burst of music meant I was dragged round the dancefloor again.

Enter the oncologist. She comes round the curtain – I am insisting that the curtain round my bed remains drawn – says, 'That's not as bad as I thought it was going to be,' and laughs. I cry. She tells me about the protocols for rejoining the drug trial. I ignore her. She goes away.

The next day, I was discharged from the hospital, and took my gradually deflating face home. It took a couple of weeks to return to normal, and a couple more for me to process what had happened. Alan thought I'd struggled because I was unprepared, and he may have been right.

BAH! THINKING

A meditation for when you are ambushed

Get comfortable. Get quiet. Breathe slowly. Count your breaths, up to 10 then back again. When your mind is still, turn your attention to your heart, your solar plexus, your head, or wherever it is that you feel that you – your essence, spirit, soul, personality – live.

Bring all of your attention to that place. (You might choose to imagine yourself as tiny and walking around inside your own heart.) Experience what being you means. It might be a feeling, or a picture, a colour, or a series of words. Think about the best of you. Think about what has been you since the earliest time.

Be taken over by that feeling of you-ness. Feel it expand your lungs and fill your limbs.

When you are ready, open your eyes. Go about your life. But remember how it feels to be you.

MONDAY, 6 JULY 2009 [ABRIDGED]: ITCHY AND SCRATCHY

Aaargh! Being itchy all the time is torture! The rash is less angry looking, but itchy as can be, and my meditation and self control has come on in leaps and bounds over the last couple of days through the sheer effort of not gouging my skin off with my fingernails. (Except (a) for 'meditation and self control' read 'knitting' as keeping my hands otherwise occupied was all I could do, and (b) I kept waking up in the night because I was scratching in my sleep…)

It's now over a week since this little ol' drama began, and I'm inclined to agree with Debby […] – it's difficult to know what is causing what after a certain point. We know that lapatinib (the trial drug) started the whole thing off. But since then I've had antihistamine, intravenously and orally, and steroid, intravenously and orally…. as well as painkillers, sleeping tablets, Tamoxifen and my usual daily thyroxine. And that's only what's going in… not what my body is adding to the mix in what I can only imagine are increasingly desperate attempts to keep some sort of a lid on it all…. it's a wonder I'm functioning at all, really! I'm trying to eat well, drink a lot of water, and knit well, all strategies for recovery before too long. After a week without an uninterrupted night's sleep (yes, I hear that hollow laughter from mums of little ones everywhere) I'm in sore need of that recovery!

It's back to the oncologist today (I am taking Alan for moral support/general defence/note taking/salient question asking) so we'll see what she has to say about it all. Not a lot, if previous visits are anything to go by, but we'll see…. One of the reasons for the appointment is to 'discuss' whether or not I'm going back on the drug trial (time allocated: 2 seconds) and another is to talk about alternative treatments. In my case this means herceptin intravenously every three weeks for a year.

🌱 🌱 🌱

Herceptin: Plan B

PLAN B

As the ALLTO trial hadn't worked out, it was on to Plan B: a year of herceptin, as standard. I wasn't enthused. I thought I'd left the hospital part of my dance with cancer behind me, but instead it was back to the chemotherapy unit, back to the search for a usable vein in my usable arm. My feelings careered endlessly round a series of fixed points when I let them, and it took a while to get a grip. There was resentment at a treatment I didn't, in my heart, feel I needed; gratitude that such drugs were available to me; general grumpiness about the hassle and time treatment took; utter remorse when I looked around the unit and saw how ill others were, and thought about how they'd take my place in a closely-monitored heartbeat.

The first time I had herceptin, I had to stay in the unit for six hours afterwards to check for allergic reactions, which can be quick and nasty and need fast treatment with intravenous antihistamines. Ned came along and the day passed uneventfully. I was deemed to be able to tolerate herceptin, and I went home. In a grump.

The next few days were low-level achy, slightly fluey, but largely OK. I thought that I would just knuckle down and get on with herceptin. And I did. For a while.

TUESDAY, 21 JULY 2009 [ABRIDGED]: GLORIOUSLY UNREMARKABLE

I'd be lying if I said I bounced out of bed this morning saying, 'Hurrah! Time for herceptin the wonder drug! What a lucky bunny I am!' [...] Still, off I went like a sensible girl, with a book, knitting, and Ned in tow to keep me occupied. (I wore the new top I bought yesterday. Something a little bit wenchy to wear always cheers me up.)

[...] we began with the ritual Heating Of The Arm in the hope that a vein might be tempted out of hiding [...] By 11.30 we were off. The herceptin goes in via a drip – it's in a saline solution – over an hour and a half. There's a meter which keeps the pace steady.

We were briefed to look out for chills, aches and any other oddnesses. I got bored with waiting to feel weird fairly quickly, and got on with [some knitting ...] Ned and I chatted, we talked to other people having treatment, and an hour and a half flew by. Herceptin 1 – done!

Because this was my first time, I had to stay on for a bit just in case I reacted. (Estimates had varied from a manageable 2 to a mind melting 8 hours.) Lovely Amy took pity on me at 4pm and let me go, I met up with Alan (who was taking over from Ned doing Stephanie-minding) and we came home.

I'm happy to report that the whole thing has been utterly unremarkable.

[...] The worst side effect is the headache brought on by 6 solid hours of enforced listening to Magic FM. (James Blunt. Mariah Carey. Two words. Enough, already.)

BAH! THINKING

Coping with hospital time

Here are some things you could do while you are in hospital for the day, not feeling unwell.

1. Read. But read something (a) easy, because you're going to get interrupted a lot, and (b) funny or uplifting, because frankly, if you want doom and gloom all you have to do is raise your eyes from the page and look around. Give yourself a break.

2. Go for a walk. There's not really any reason why you shouldn't, and wheeling your drip stand around with you does have a certain novelty value, especially if you meet someone else equally inexperienced with a drip stand coming the other way.

3. Save yourself a few big crosswords and work through them as you sit.

4. If you have company, take a pack of cards, and re-acquaint yourself with rummy or learn poker. Even Snap! is more fun than looking at each other while you both wonder whether you are having an adverse reaction or not.

5.   Knit. Or crochet. Not only is this a great thing to do in its own right, but if you are knitting, people will watch you, and chat to you, and ask what you are doing, and tell you about their hobbies, and before you know it a couple of hours will have grown on your needles.

6.   If you don't want to be social, take an iPod with something good and long on it. An opera, a film, the complete works of The Beatles, your favourite book read by your favourite actor ... It doesn't matter what it is, so long as it transforms three hours of being stuck in a chair into three hours of indulgence.

7.   Take someone you don't see enough of, and catch up.

WEDNESDAY, 23 DECEMBER 2009 [ABRIDGED]: HERCEPTIN FAILS TO HAPPEN

Herceptin day dawned once more today. I wasn't in the best of moods, but I never am on herceptin day. I had a little cry before Alan and I set off for the hospital, but I sometimes do. We arrived, and we chatted to a lady that we often see in the waiting room, and I was called after 40 minutes [...] – and up until then it was all pretty much as normal.

The first attempt to cannulate failed. Again, not unusual. But the amount of pain involved in the failed cannulation seemed greater than it usually is. (When the needle finds the vein, after the initial scratch it doesn't hurt. When the needle misses, that means it's scratching around in your tissues, and that does.) So – the next unusual thing – as Joanna got ready for another attempt,

I started to cry. Not lace-edged hanky crying, either. I felt it well up from somewhere very deep, and once it started, it wasn't stopping. The fact that I felt a wimp and an idiot didn't help slow things down. The fact that being treated near me were two people who looked as though they had been through more in the last week than I had been through in the last year made me try really hard to stop crying, and I was doing that thing that toddlers do, you know, when it all goes quiet for a minute or two and you think 'right, she's stopped' but actually she's just getting set for the next bawl? That was me. Joanna took us into the Quiet Room (which wasn't quiet for long) and was kind and comforting, and I kept trying to calm down, and failing. Then Joanna left us alone and I hit the crying-too-much-to-breathe stage, and that gave me enough of a fright that I got a hold on things. A bit.

Joanna came back and told me off (in a lovely way) for (a) apologising and (b) saying I was OK. We talked about what to do. I asked if she would have a go at cannulating in the Quiet Room, so she went off to get the trolley, and I kept trying to talk myself calm, kept at it with the breathing techniques and the self hypnosis, but it was no good; the tears just kept coming.

Joanna spent a long time trying to find a good vein, but here's the problem, step by step:

1. My veins were never great to start with.

2. Chemotherapy damages the veins, so what started bad has got worse.

3. Only my left arm can be used, as I have had lymph nodes removed on the right side.

4.   There were three visible, usable veins until 6 weeks ago, when the vein that was tried was severely bruised and has never recovered – it remains black-and-blue. So, 2 possibilities. Each can be tried more than once, so long as you start near the hand and work up.

5.   Although herceptin doesn't damage veins the way that chemo does, every time a needle is inserted, or there's an attempt to insert a needle, a little bit of scar tissue is created, and that scar tissue makes it more difficult to get into the vein.

So, we weren't starting from a good place.

I've had this done so often now that I can tell when the nurses have found a part of the vein that's going to work. When they press against the point they are going to put the needle into, the vein sort of springs back, just like a sponge cake does when it is ready to come out of the oven. And as Joanna pressed and probed, there was nothing springing back at all. So I asked her to stop, and we waited for Manjula, Cannula Queen, to come back from lunch and have a go.

She had two goes. Again, no springing back. Both attempts really, properly hurt. Both failed. I cried throughout, and felt terrible about it. We talked about what to do next, and Manjula arranged for us to go to another ward, where the team cannulate using ultrasound to find veins that aren't easily visible. We were all mindful, as we talked, of the fact that I need to have herceptin another 11 times, and this is when I said the words I thought I'd never say: that maybe I needed to have a PICC line again. (In order to prevent Alan from falling off his chair and fracturing something

I did actually say, 'I can't believe I am about to say this,' before I said it. He did wobble, but he didn't fall. His face was a picture.)

Anyway. We had half an hour to go until we could be seen in the other ward, so we went for a coffee. I was still crying. All I wanted to do was get out of there. After a bit of discussion we decided that that's what we would do. Alan went back up to the Trevor Howell unit to tell the team that he was taking me home, and had a chat with Rachael where they agreed that (a) this was the best thing to do, (b) that the tooth situation couldn't be helping and Rachael would renew her efforts to help me to be seen by the people in charge of door handles and string.

So that's what we did. (Via Sainsbury's, where we did the Christmas food shopping and escaped pretty unscathed and with everything we wanted, bar a few judicious substitutions for what they'd run out of.) I didn't have my herceptin, and right now I feel as though I don't want to have any more, and I don't want to have a PICC line again, and I never want anyone to come near me with a needle ever ever again, and I certainly never want to set foot in St George's ever ever ever again (except to have my tooth out, when I will ride there naked on a llama through the snow if that's what I have to do to get rid of the wretched thing).

I have no idea why everything hit me so hard today, but it did. It wasn't really about the needles. It was about the difficulty of going back every three weeks when I really want to be done with cancer. It was about being reminded of this time last year when I was getting ready for chemotherapy and had no idea of what was to come. It was about the way that, because herceptin is 'not as bad as chemotherapy', it gets a bit forgotten and a bit not bothered about by everyone, including the oncology team. It was about being in pain all the time, and tired all the time, and overshadowed by treatment all the time. It was about not looking on the bright side, not keeping my chin up, not being strong. I felt frightened. I felt out of control.

But I also felt supported and looked after. No one (except me) told me not to be silly or to get over it.

IT ALL STARTS TO GET A BIT MUCH

Whereas the ALLTO trial had gone spectacularly wrong, herceptin didn't. Herceptin went a little bit wrong in many, many ways.

It wasn't long until finding a vein became more and more problematic, and so, as you know, the PICC came back.

The 'mild flu-like symptoms' that oncologists cite as a side effect – but in a way that makes it sound like a Special Treat because you're Doing So Well – were lousy. If you've ever had actual flu, you'll know that feeling the day before the shivering and burning sets in. It's the day when things that should be easy, like making a cup of tea, answering the phone, or deciding what to wear, seem insurmountable and exhausting. It's the day when you have a low-level ache in every part of you, even your toenails and your earlobes and your blood. Well, I had that for four days after every treatment.

There were other little things, too. The inside of my nose dried and scabbed and hurt all the time. (After a little advice from a nurse, I never went anywhere without Vaseline, and became expert at coating the insides of my nostrils with it half a dozen times a day. Try it. It's not as easy as it sounds. But possibly more revolting than it sounds. Bag balm – used by farmers on cows with chapping on their udders – works well, too.) And I ached. I was stiff and sore when I got up in the morning, and felt like a cartoon grandma as I made my way painfully downstairs each morning. One of my CT scans showed my heart to be dangerously underperforming, and although the repeat heart exam a week later showed it as being normal again, I got a fright.

All of these minor symptoms started to become a major weight. Despite giving myself a daily talking-to, using herceptin aftermath days as an excuse to watch some boxed DVD sets, read and knit a lot, counting my blessings and reminding myself that it Wasn't Long Now and I was, in fact, Very Lucky To Be Alive and to have the opportunity to have this drug, I struggled.

I will admit I spent a lot of time behaving like a five-year-old who doesn't want to eat up her broccoli, but wobbly bottom lip aside, I could tell that with every cycle of herceptin I was becoming a little lower, and not being able to quite pick myself up before the next one began. It was like running laps, but every lap getting just a fraction longer, without there being any more time to get round the circuit. (I'm hypothesizing. I don't do running.)

I was just past the halfway point of herceptin, nine of 18 treatments and a cool £27,000 worth of drugs, when the PICC line became infected. It burned and wept and when we took it down to the hospital one Sunday morning, the duty oncologist had it taken out as soon as she looked at it. And as the oncologist prescribed some hefty antibiotics, I confessed that I was wondering whether I wanted to continue with herceptin, I braced myself for Oncologist Chat 24b – 'I know it's hard now but you will recover and you can take paracetamol and in six months it will all be over and anyway shouldn't you be grateful and glad to be alive and thinking of your children not yourself' – but what I actually got was, 'Well, we have to give you a year of herceptin because that's the standard of care, but there's increasing evidence to show that we over-prescribe it.'

Alan and I talked and did some research (well, I typed 'duration of herceptin' into Google) and pondered, and couldn't really make up our minds what to do. So we did this.

de Bono's Six Thinking Hats®

We've mentioned all of the Hats individually now – White Hat for data, Red Hat for instinct, Green Hat for new ideas, Black Hat for risks, Yellow Hat for benefits, and Blue Hat for managing the process. Each Hat is useful in itself – but the real power comes when you put them together. This is a 'parallel thinking' system, and because everyone wears the same Hat at the same time, there's no debate or argument. Because you wear all of the Hats, you're forced to see the subject from every point of view. Organizations I've worked with using the Six Hats have seen meeting times drop by 50 per cent, no lengthy debate or getting off-topic, more robust decisions and sorting out complex problems. In this case, it was this last benefit we were interested in.

MONDAY, 22 MARCH 2010 [ABRIDGED]: THE MINUTES OF THE MEETING

Cue secret weapon: it was time to get the Six Thinking Hats® out.

[...] So, over the remains of brunch in Reds Bar and Grill in Wimbledon, Alan and I did some structured thinking. Here's what we came up with. As so often happens with the Hats, we got further in 20 minutes than we did in the last three weeks.

Red Hat: what is our gut instinct about continuing with herceptin?

Uncertain, x 2.

White Hat: what information do we have?

The cancer has been removed in its entirety, as far as anyone can tell

I've had 2 (chemotherapy, radiotherapy) and a half (9 rounds of herceptin) 'insurance policies' against it returning [...]

I have continual but varying side effects, which include: joint aches, muscle cramps, heart flutterings, chest pain, constantly sore and bleeding nose, and nausea. (Oh, and I sleep badly, but looking at that list, it's hardly surprising, is it?!)

Side effects have been getting progressively worse, as I have not fully recovered from one dose before I have the next

Roche, the manufacturers of herceptin, recommend that it should be prescribed for a year

A Finnish study has shown 9 weeks of herceptin to be as effective as a year

The on-call oncologist who had my infected PICC removed said there is evidence to suggest that too much herceptin is given

Herceptin has been shown to deliver great results, especially when give concurrently with chemotherapy

One study suggests that I am in the group of people least likely to benefit from herceptin – and that's women with HER2 positive, hormone positive, node negative cancers, not blondes or mothers or people who knit

I will be taking Tamoxifen for another 4 years, which takes care of the hormone-positive risk element

Yellow Hat: what are the benefits of continuing with herceptin?

We would be doing the right thing in terms of current medical thinking

If I did accidentally sprout another cancer in the future, we could be confident that we did everything we could have to prevent it

The herceptin might be stopping a new cancer from growing

I'd have something to blog about every three weeks (Alan gave me a Look when I said that. But hey, benefits is benefits.)

Black Hat: what are the risks of continuing with herceptin?

There could be a continuing decline in my physical health and in my mental wellbeing if the process continues to drain my resources as it's doing now

I'd need a new means of delivery, such as a PICC or Hickman line, which means discomfort, limitations and infection risk

The treatment may be completely unnecessary, if there is no cancer for it to prevent

The treatment is time consuming and hospital visits are frustrating

We would face another 6 months of worry and stress around side effects

It would be 6 months before we, as a family, could put this behind us

Treatment is a drain on everyone, not just me, so we'd have another 6 months of that

Green Hat: how could we overcome those Black Hat difficulties?

We could design a structured programme of interventions and therapies for me – hypnotherapy, yoga, counselling, etc. – which would happen throughout treatment rather than waiting for crisis points

We could ask about a PowerPort or have the PICC sited somewhere where there would be less risk of infection

We could ask about having the treatment accelerated and book other hospital appointments in on herceptin days

We could start looking forward to what we will be doing in 6 months and onward to help us to focus on then rather than now

We could ask the oncologist what s/he can tell us about current research and current oncological (?) thinking about herceptin

We could involve more people in my welfare and ask for more help from friends and family in terms of helping me to cope with side effects and keeping my spirits up

Red Hat: having looked at this, how do we now feel about continuing herceptin?

Alan: still don't know, but feel better equipped to deal with it either way

Me: happy to go on if necessary

Blue Hat: what are the next steps?

List questions for oncologist and go to appointment tomorrow open-minded and aware that we don't have enough information to make the decision

If we do decide to go ahead with herceptin, put our Green Hat ideas into action immediately

So, there you have it. I feel much better now: much more comfortable that, whatever the decision is, we will handle it and it will be OK. We have knowledge, we have questions, we have plans.

We'll be OK.

So, we met with an oncologist to talk about stopping herceptin. She didn't fall off her chair in horror at the idea. She didn't seem very surprised at all. She said it was our decision and then she told us that, had I been diagnosed later, she would have been recommending me for the Persephone trial, which was looking at six months versus 12 months of herceptin. So had I been on the Persephone trial, I might have been given six months of herceptin as my whole treatment.

That was the critical piece of White Hat data that we were missing.

We went away, we thought and talked and went through the Hats again, and then we rang the hospital and said that I wasn't going to be having any more herceptin.

I've always felt I made the right decision; but I didn't feel any relief or excitement or big WooHoo! as I put the phone down after making the call. I took some painkillers and went to sleep for the afternoon. I slept better than I had done in months.

BAH! THINKING

Questions for your oncology team if you're not happy

In the end, it was getting enough White Hat data that helped us to think our way through herceptin and its difficulties. Here are some good questions to start with.

1. Why is this drug prescribed for this amount of time?

2. Why do you think this is a suitable drug for me?

3. Do you know of any studies that are looking at the duration of treatment with this drug?

4. Have you had any other patients who have chosen to take this drug for a shorter amount of time?

5. What are the implications of stopping taking this drug?

6. What else can you do to help with the side effects of this drug?

7. Are there any alternatives to this drug?

BAH! THINKING
Whine time

When herceptin side effects were really getting me down, I invented something that I called Whine Time. I allocated myself a maximum of 10 minutes per day, divided into no more than two sessions. For that time, I was allowed to whine. But the point was to get it out of my system somehow, so I didn't allow myself to just think whiny thoughts. I had to either write them down or say them out loud. Here are some of the ways I whined. Feel free to use them yourself.

1. I talked to Alan, Ned or Joy, or sometimes all three.

2. I rang Mum.

3. I rang Dad.

4. I wrote a whiney blog post.

5. I wrote 'aaargh!' over and over again on a piece of paper, then I put it in the bin.

6. I wrote a list of everything I hated about herceptin treatment.

7. I got into the shower and sang, 'I am sick of herceptin,' to the tune of 'I Will Always Love You.'

8. I stroked the cat and complained at her.

9. I called a friend and said, 'Let me whinge for 10 minutes but then make me talk about something else.'

10. I lay on my bed and hit the pillows and cried. And I stopped quite soon because that feels really silly, unless you're in a film.

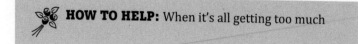

HOW TO HELP: When it's all getting too much

If your loved one is suffering, it's easy to try to jolly them along, and that sometimes works, but that's not always the right thing to do. Here are some other strategies:

1.   Ask a lot of questions. Try to find out exactly what's wrong. Ask: Where does it hurt? What sort of pain? How long does it last? What makes it worse? Getting the true picture will help you both when it comes to explaining what's happening to someone else.

2.   Suggest, and make, appointments with people who can help. That might be the oncologist, to discuss treatment, or it might be that a sympathetic GP is the best first port of call. The important thing is not to let the situation continue; if your loved one is low, they may lack the motivation to do anything about the problem. Do it for them.

3.   Go along to appointments.

4.   Don't assume that the view you get from the medical professional you are talking to is the only view. It may be; it may not. Do your own research, too. Ask for a second opinion.

5.   When you go anywhere with your loved one, take tissues and painkillers.

6.   Most importantly of all: listen. Really listen.

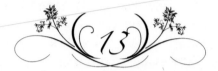

Tamoxifen: I feel it in my fingers, I feel it in my toes

TUESDAY, 12 MAY 2009 [ABRIDGED]: A NEW REGIME

This morning, I took Tamoxifen for the first time. I'm going to be … [doing] this … every morning for at least the next 5 years. (The current view is that 5 years of Tamoxifen is plenty, but new studies are starting to show that longer might be even better.)

Tamoxifen is a drug that blocks the body's ability to absorb oestrogen. As oestrogen is one of the things that the particular type of breast cancer I had feeds on, this drug simply makes it very difficult for any cancer cells there might be hanging around to grow.

As you know if you're a regular reader, Stephanie's Official View On Whether There Is Any Cancer Left In Her Body can be summed up in two words: there isn't. But that doesn't mean I'm not going to take out yet more insurance against a return.

The possible side effects of Tamoxifen include the usual suspects: tiredness, nausea, aches and pains. Then there are the early menopausal symptoms, but that's really only going to be finishing what the chemotherapy started. Cervical cancer is less likely but a possibility – you couldn't make it up, could you?! However the chances of these side effects vary from slim to skeletal, so I am going to assume the best, carry on exactly as though I have no side effects whatsoever, and expect my body to follow suit.

ABOUT TAMOXIFEN

Tamoxifen is the other element in the 'starve cancer' strategy. Herceptin stops the body's uptake of HER2; Tamoxifen stops the uptake of oestrogen.

The big benefit of Tamoxifen – aside from the whole cancer-prevention thing – is that it comes in tablet form. A little round sugar-coated tablet, a bit like a Smartie or an M&M, and as easily swallowed. It doesn't disrupt your life. It just slips down, every day, for five years, starting as soon as chemotherapy stops.

There are two big drawbacks of Tamoxifen:

1.   Medical menopause.

2.   Swollen feet and hands.

Let's take the menopause first. Tamoxifen stops your body from absorbing oestrogen, the hormone that makes women fertile, and makes us menstruate if we aren't pregnant. The natural menopause happens when the body naturally and slowly stops producing oestrogen. Medical menopause is more abrupt. The symptoms are pretty much the same, though: night sweats, stopped periods, hot flushes, dry skin, mood swings, weight gain ... although I decided that the last two were optional and did my best not to have them.

I have mixed feelings about the medical menopause. I think all of these thoughts, often all at the same time:

- If I'm going to have a menopause I may as well get it over with when there's so much else going on – radiotherapy, herceptin, general dealing-with-cancer-and-fallout – and I won't get caught up in it.

- It's quite nice not to have to faff around with periods and pre-menstrual tension.

- Why has the medical profession assumed that I don't want to have any more children?

- It's. Not. Fair.

- This dance with cancer seems designed to rob me of my femininity – ugly breasts and sterile at 38.

- I had no intentions of having any more children, and I'm alive, so it doesn't matter at all.

I think this is a really good example of how cancer can re-calibrate your idea of what matters and what doesn't. Had I experienced an early natural menopause as a healthy 38 year old, I'm fairly sure I would have been devastated (and a lot more moody). But as it happened, after all of the needles and hair loss and illness, a medical menopause wasn't really much to add. A bit like spraining your ankle when you already have both arms in plaster and a patch over your eye.

(What is a little bit infuriating, though, is the possibility that I might start menstruating again at 43 when I stop taking Tamoxifen, and then get to do the menopause once more, in the traditional way. I may allow myself to be moody when that happens.)

BAH! THINKING

A daily meditation for daily medication

Sit still. Sit comfortably. Hold the tablet in your hand. Allow yourself to become quiet inside.

When you are ready, swallow the tablet.

Close your eyes and imagine the tablet travelling into your stomach. Imagine it dissolving and making its way around your body. Imagine it doing what it needs to do.

Welcome it.

Feel how protected you are.

Smile.

Open your eyes and go about your day.

The second big side effect of Tamoxifen is swelling in the hands and feet, which is in the category of 'side effects that oncologists mention in passing because they aren't medically significant but actually have a really big impact'. Within six months of starting Tamoxifen, I was in a jeweller's having my wedding and engagement rings cut off because they were wedged onto my finger. I developed an ingrowing toenail because my shoes became tighter and tighter, until

I realized what was happening and started buying size 9 instead of size 8. My habitual style of dressing – pretty skirts or dresses, tights and heels – has had to give way to trousers and flat sandals in summer, dresses and boots in winter, because I am self-conscious about my bulging ankles. But these things are not, I know, the end of the world. Alan and I had a new wedding ring made. I knit pretty socks as a way of loving my feet (and not having to look at them).

BAH! THINKING

Some approaches to swelling, bulging, and gaining weight

Maybe weight gain isn't important to you – or maybe you have a skinny rather than a fat cancer. But if you do gain weight, bulge or swell as a result of treatment (or, in my case, custard), here are some things to think about doing.

1. Decide whether weight gain is going to be something permanent or something that you will live with for a while then deal with. (I ate custard and drank chocolate milk to ease the vicious heartburn that came with chemotherapy. I knew it was making me gain weight but, at the time, dealing with the symptom mattered more. I lost the weight later, when the heartburn was over.)

2. If you're living with it forever, get rid of clothes that stop fitting as they stop fitting. Replace them with well-fitting, good-looking clothes. Being big doesn't mean tracksuit bottoms and men's T-shirts, unless you want it to.

3. If weight gain is a short-term side effect, buy a couple of outfits that fit well, in a bigger size. You will look and feel better in a size 16 that fits than in a size 14 that you are oozing out of.

4. Ask people you trust what your best features are. Emphasize them.

5. Remember that if you lose your hair your head will look smaller and therefore your body will seem bigger. Find hats that have a bit of body, like berets or hats with brims, and pleat headscarves at the front before you tie them.

6. Recognize what aspect of your body makes you most uncomfortable and deal with that. (I stopped wearing anything that revealed my ankles in summer, because every time I looked at my poor swollen feet and ankles it made me want to cry.)

7. Recognize also that you are likely to be more critical of yourself than anyone else is. I'm pretty sure that if I did go out in a knee-length skirt, my friends wouldn't all be texting each other horrified texts about the state of my legs.

14

Moving on:
The same, but different

LITTLE DID I KNOW

When I told Ned and Joy that I had a cancer, I told them something else too. I said, 'Absolutely nothing around here is going to change.' Ned still teases me about it. But at the time – I remember this – I believed it. Fervently. I believed that the best possible thing I could do for my children was to be The Same and to Keep Going and to Be Brave and to Just Get On With It. I saw myself, I think, as a cross between a dinner lady and one of those obscure female saints martyred by having their breasts hacked off.

As I write this final chapter, less than two years after diagnosis, I almost don't know how to begin explaining what my dance with cancer has done to me and to my life. It would be easy to slip into one of those 'Hello trees, hello sky, live every moment as though it's your last'-type endings, but it's not really that simple. Or that twee. The best way I can think of to explain what has happened to me is by likening it to the tempering of metal. The heat burns all of the impurities away, and what's left is strong and bright and better. Dancing with cancer challenged me to look at my life and myself and to get rid of what shouldn't be there. I'm not saying that I'm perfect now: I'm far from it. But I have learned and changed and I hope that, now I've got the hang of learning and changing, I will keep doing it, so that one day I will be worthy of all of the love and time that my family, friends, assorted strangers, and the medical profession, have invested in keeping me walking this good Earth.

MONDAY, 6 JULY 2009 [ABRIDGED]: THE BLUE SKY CLUB

When this whole dance with cancer began, there were a lot of people I had to tell quickly, and I tried to tell them in person or at least speak to them on the phone. One person I couldn't do that with, though, was my colleague and friend Rob, who was at a conference in Tokyo at the time, with a different time zone and a phone that wasn't taking calls from the UK … so I had to send him an email. (There were pressing work reasons why I couldn't wait until he got back.)

The reply I got was supportive and positive and lovely. It included this:

"I am so sorry to hear this news, but having had my Dad go through colonic cancer some 15–20 years ago, I can only say that your thinking this is not a big deal is definitely the BEST way to approach this. My Dad still takes the view that a lot of the damage can be self inflicted and that mind over matter is by far the best way to approach this. It worked for him, when he was given 4–6 weeks to live, and made a full recovery."

On Saturday, we celebrated Rob's 40th birthday at a terrific party, and I was lucky enough to meet Rob's parents. His dad shook my hand and welcomed me to The Blue Sky Club. No, I'd never heard of it either, and that's because Rob's dad invented it the day he came out of hospital, looked up, and thought 'Ah! Blue sky! How wonderful!' The Blue Sky Club is a lovely way of encapsulating the idea that your life can be changed irrevocably for the better by a dance with cancer.

I don't know Rob's dad very well, but I've known Rob for 5 years now, and it's clear that he too is a fully paid up member of the Blue Sky Club. He appreciates his friends, values his colleagues and clients, and is utterly devoted to his family. He has built a company that delivers with passion and integrity. And he's always fundraising. (Just in case you want to run and hide from this tedious paragon... he's also great fun.) Now I'm sure Rob would always have turned out to be a decent guy. But I suspect that his dad's dance with cancer, and membership of the Blue Sky Club, has been a huge influence.

So as well as having a lovely time at a great party, I came away inspired by Rob's dad and reassured that this dance with cancer might have changed the lives of me and mine in more positive ways that I'd dared to imagine [...]

Yes, I'm a member of the Blue Sky Club. Are you?

de Bono's PMI

PMI stands for 'Plus, Minus, Interesting'. It's a way of quickly assessing something without getting carried away by feelings or perception. A PMI on the outcomes of my dance with cancer might go something like this:

Plus

- I've learned that I don't have to be responsible for everything.

- My relationships with my husband, my family and most of my friends are stronger.

- I've dropped things that I wasn't enjoying from my life and focus on what gives me pleasure.

- I've got really good at knitting.

- I have remembered how much I love to write, and learned to write in a way that helps and, sometimes, heals.

- I've moved to a new home in a beautiful place.

- I'm getting better at accepting help.

- At the centre of me now is a grain of golden calm that never goes.

Minus

- My body hasn't really recovered. I now have the worst nails and the feeblest digestive system you can imagine. And it took three months for a mosquito bite to heal in the summer.

- There are times when the fear of having to go through it all again traps me like a moth in amber.

- I hated watching people I love be afraid for me and upset as I suffered.

- For some people I will always now be defined as someone who had breast cancer.

- There were some friends who turned out to be not such good friends after all.

- There are pictures of my breasts on the internet (and they are the kind of breasts that only a ravenous newborn could love).

Interesting

- Although I am choosing to be public about my dance with cancer, not sure how I feel about being labelled a cancer survivor.

- Sometimes I mourn for my pre-cancer self, for her reckless good health and assumption that the sun would always shine.

- Sometimes I feel sorry for her, racing around never thinking about whether she was doing what she really needed and wanted to be doing, in need of something to give her a fresh interpretation of her days.

All of this begs the question: if I had the option to go back and dance with cancer or not dance with cancer, what would I do? And the honest answer is: I don't know. It was foul and I would give anything not to have had to put myself and my beloveds through it (and that's bearing in mind that I am one of the lucky ones who is here to tell the tale). And yet, and yet ... I have a sneaking suspicion that owing to my dance with cancer, the rest of my life will be happier and more fulfilled and fulfilling than it would otherwise have been.

BAH! THINKING 🦅

A meditation for moving on

I do this every night before I go to sleep.

Get comfortable. Breathe slowly. Make sure you are still and warm. Breathe deep, slow, breaths that expand your stomach and fill your lungs. Breathe twice as slowly as you think you can.

When you are relaxed and ready, imagine every cell in your body as full of health. You might see them as being full of light, or perfectly round, or pulsing with life, or with a speck of perfect well-being at their centre. However you do it, feel wellness throughout you.

Smile.

Sleep.

Be well.

Oh, and Bah! to cancer.

Resources

CANCER BOOKS

Val Sampson and Debbie Fenlon, *The Breast Cancer Book: A Personal Guide to Help You Through It and Beyond* (Vermillion, 2002)

David Serban-Schreiber, *Anticancer: A New Way of Life* (Michael Joseph, 2008)

Dr Bernie Siegel, *Love, Medicine and Miracles* (Rider, 1999)

CANCER INFORMATION WEBSITES

www.cancerhelp.org.uk

www.macmillan.org.uk

DR EDWARD DE BONO

Six Thinking Hats (Penguin, 2009)

How to Have a Beautiful Mind (Vermilion, 2004)

www.debonothinkingsystems.com

www.sixhatthinking.co.uk

www.indigobusiness.co.uk

THINKING, MEDITATION AND VISUALIZATION

Shakti Gawain, *Meditations: Creative Visualisation and Meditation Exercises to Enrich Your Life* (New World Library, 2003)

Eric Harrison, *Teach Yourself to Meditate: Over 20 Exercises for Peace, Health and Clarity of Mind* (Piatkus, 1994)

Professor Richard Wiseman, *59 Seconds: Think a little, change a lot* (Pan, 2010)

www.gosiagorna.com

Hay House Titles of Related Interest

Cancer (CD), *by Louise L. Hay*

Eliminating Stress, Finding Inner Peace
(book with CD), by Brian L. Weiss

Heal Your Body, *by Louise L. Hay*

Help Me to Heal, *by Bernie S. Siegel*

How Your Mind Can Heal Your Body,
by David R. Hamilton PhD

The Power of Joy (CD),
by Dr Christiane Northrup

You Can Heal Your Life, *by Louise L. Hay*

JOIN THE HAY HOUSE FAMILY

As the leading self-help, mind, body and spirit publisher in the UK, we'd like to welcome you to our family so that you can enjoy all the benefits our website has to offer.

 EXTRACTS from a selection of your favourite author titles

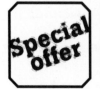 **COMPETITIONS, PRIZES & SPECIAL OFFERS** Win extracts, money off, downloads and so much more

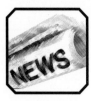 **LISTEN** to a range of radio interviews and our latest audio publications

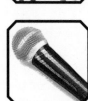 **CELEBRATE YOUR BIRTHDAY** An inspiring gift will be sent your way

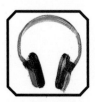 **LATEST NEWS** Keep up with the latest news from and about our authors

 ATTEND OUR AUTHOR EVENTS Be the first to hear about our author events

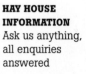 **iPHONE APPS** Download your favourite app for your iPhone

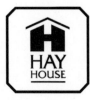 **HAY HOUSE INFORMATION** Ask us anything, all enquiries answered

join us online at **www.hayhouse.co.uk**

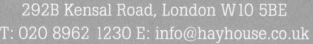
292B Kensal Road, London W10 5BE
T: 020 8962 1230 E: info@hayhouse.co.uk

ABOUT THE AUTHOR

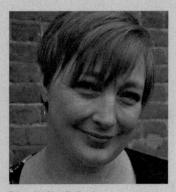

Stephanie Butland was diagnosed with a breast cancer in October 2008. Since then she's had surgery, chemotherapy, radiotherapy and drug treatment, and now she's thriving. She lives in rural Northumberland with her family, near the place where she grew up, close to beaches, an ice cream parlour, and most of her family. (It would be heaven if it was a little bit warmer.) Her move 'back home' after 20 years of living in London was one of the very positive side-effects of her dance with cancer.

Taken by Alan Butland

Stephanie writes in her studio, which sits under the branches of an apple tree at the bottom of her garden. Between books and articles, she blogs and speaks about surviving cancer. Her aims are simple: to show that breast cancer is not necessarily the end of the world, and to try to make a dance with cancer easier for others by sharing the approaches and strategies that worked for her.

When she's not writing, Stephanie coaches thinking skills and creativity throughout Europe, and works with individuals to help them to think more effectively. In her spare time, she knits, spins, reads, bakes, goes to the theatre, takes long walks on quiet beaches, and makes excellent use of any shopping opportunity that comes her way.

You'll find Stephanie's blog, and more information about her and her work, at www.bahtocancer.com

www.bahtocancer.com